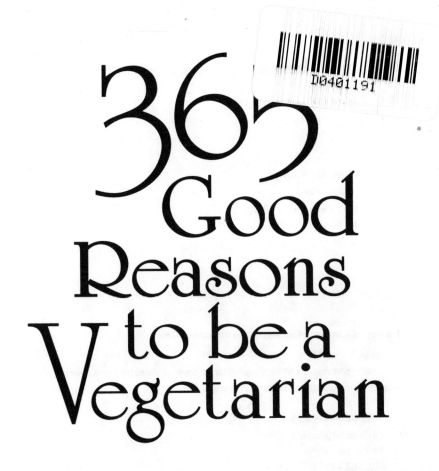

365 Good Reasons to be a Vegetarian

Victor Parachin

Avery Publishing Group
Garden City Park, New York

Cover Design: William Gonzalez and Rudy Shur
Typesetting: Rhonda Wincek
Text Illustrator: John Wincek
In-House Editor: Dara Stewart

Avery Publishing Group
120 Old Broadway
Garden City Park, NY 11040
1-800-548-5757

Library of Congress Cataloging-in-Publication Data
Parachin, Victor M.
   365 good reasons to be a vegetarian: a book of thoughts, facts, humor,
science, and surprises / Victor M. Parachin.
     p. cm
    ISBN 0-89529-813-9
    1. Vegetarianism. I. Title.
   TX392.p35 1997
   613.2'62—dc21   97-46060
                                           CIP

Printed in the United States of America

10 9 8 7 6 5 4 3 2 1

With love to my mother, Val,
whose interest in nutrition and health
was ahead of its time.

Acknowledgments

No book is ever the sole result of the author alone. I am no exception and would like to thank sincerely the following individuals:

Rudy Shur, managing editor of Avery Publishing Group, who believed in this book from the beginning and whose editorial insights and judgments sharpened the focus and improved the overall quality of my writing;

The editors and writers at the *Vegetarian Resource Group*, *Vegetarian Times*, and *Veggie Life*—their articles and recipes continue to inspire and amaze me;

The reference librarians at the Pomona (California) Public Library, who are always eager and enthusiastic in their assistance.

Introduction

"Pythagoras . . . entirely abstained from wine and animal food
. . . and confined himself to such nutriments as was slender and
easy of digestion. In consequence of this, his sleep was short,
and his soul vigilant, and pure, and his body confirmed in a state
of perfect and invariable health."

—*T. Taylor, Life of Pythagoras*

Vegetarianism is on the rise. Although vegetarianism has been
widely practiced and is the norm in many cultures around the
world, the wealthy, industrialized peoples of the West have been
voracious meat consumers. Currently, that is changing dramatically. Millions are turning away from flesh foods. In Great
Britain, 7 percent of the population (some 3 million Britons) are
vegetarians. In the United States, the number of vegetarians continues to climb, from 8 million in the 1980s to 14 million in the
1990s. Today, the real question is no longer, "Why become a
vegetarian?" but rather "Why eat meat?".

This book is written for people who are currently vegetarians,
for those who are seriously considering becoming vegetarians,
and for those who are mildly curious about a vegetarian diet.
Although I cite 365 reasons for being a vegetarian, all of them are
connected to three basic premises:

1. A vegetarian diet is healthier than a meat-based one.
2. A vegetarian diet uses natural resources (land, water, energy)
   more efficiently than does a meat-based diet.
3. A vegetarian diet does not require the suffering and death of
   animals.

It is my hope that the reasons cited for adopting a vegetarian diet (and there is one for every day of the year) will provide inspiration and information, humor and hope, and motivation and method to all who journey on the vegetarian path.

Victor M. Parachin

1 *You'll be in good company.* When many people hear the word "vegetarian," the image that suddenly appears is that of an Indian guru, complete with loincloth and skinny arms and legs. However, vegetarians are people from all walks of life. Many prominent women and men are vegetarians. Consider just these: Hank Aaron, major league baseball home run champion; Christie Brinkley, model and actress; Billie Jean King, tennis champion; Roger Brown, professional football player; Bill Pearl, four-time Mr. Universe, bodybuilder, and author; Dustin Hoffman, actor; Henry Heimlich, M.D., physician and inventor of the Heimlich maneuver; Michael Medved, film critic and author; Steve Martin, comedian and actor; Kathy Johnson, Olympic silver medalist in gymnastics; and Debbie Spaeth-Herring, Georgia State champion powerlifter. Some famous vegetarians throughout history include Leonardo Da Vinci, Thomas Edison, Albert Einstein, John Milton, Albert Schweitzer, Mary Wollstonecraft Shelley, Percy Bysshe Shelley, and John Wesley, founder of the Methodist Church.

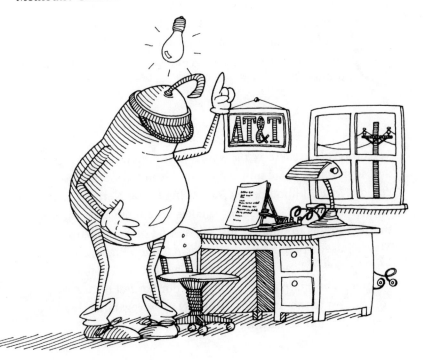

2 *It's better for your budget.* Ounce for ounce, plants and grains are thriftier choices than meat products. There is no doubt that buying potatoes, rice, beans, fruits, carrots, broccoli, tomatoes, and other vegetables is much less expensive than buying beef, chicken, and fish. The amount you save on your weekly grocery bill will allow you to splurge at an exotic vegetarian restaurant from time to time.

You will help all creatures, great and small. Many who turn to vegetarianism for dietary or health reasons soon move on to a heightened awareness of animal welfare and environmental issues. This was true for actress and bodybuilder Spice Williams. Although her vegetarian diet choice was triggered by a desire for better health, she quickly became interested in the impact on animals. "You start cleaning your body out, you become much more spiritually aware, you become closer to the environment, and you elevate yourself to a different level where it's not even about the nutritional aspect," she says. "You turn around and think, 'What are we doing killing these animals?'."

Vegetarians help conserve the world's food supply. Grains and soybeans that are now fed to American livestock could feed 1.3 billion people, according to the North American Vegetarian Society. "It takes 16 pounds of corn, wheat, or other grains to produce just one pound of meat," says Massachusetts psychologist, Charles A. Salter, Ph.D., author of *The Vegetarian Teen.* "We should realize that each person who becomes a vegetarian helps conserve our natural resources and contributes to the future of the planet. The vegetarian frees up land that could be used to help feed the less fortunate."

It's unlikely that you'll get mad cow disease. A dangerous link exists between mad cow disease—or bovine spongiform encephalopathy (BSE)—which has killed many British cattle herds, and Creutzfeld-Jakob syndrome, a fatal brain illness in humans. Humans can get Creutzfeld-Jakob syndrome by eating beef infected with BSE. The syndrome causes loss of memory and bodily control, and is incurable. The first documented case was that of Jon Resneck of Britain. His case was diagnosed in 1982, and he died three weeks after the diagnosis at the age of 28. Another documented case was that of Mary Heinz, who first complained of a total loss of sight that took place in only one night. The next day her condition deteriorated to complete loss of movement. She died the following day. Since then, many others have died from mad cow disease, which one can get only by eating contaminated beef.

A vegetarian diet combats the symptoms of menopause. Working with *Prevention Magazine,* Fredi Kronenberg, Ph.D., director of menopause research at the Center for Women's Health at Columbia-Presbyterian Medical Center in New York City, developed a questionnaire on menopause. An impressive 15,000 *Prevention* readers responded.

When women begin menopause, many experience sleep problems, hot flashes, fatigue, loss of sexual desire, mood swings, water retention, anxiety, depression, and weight gain. Vegetarian women reported fewer problems and symptoms related to menopause than did nonvegetarians. Researchers believe that the vegetarian women fared better due to the natural estrogens contained in plants. They speculate that menopausal symptoms are related to falling estrogen levels, a drop that is curtailed by increased consumption of plants and grains.

According to Socrates, you will live a peaceful and healthy life. In Plato's *Republic,* Socrates describes the ideal state to his friend Glaucon. He says the diet will be vegetarian. "For food, they will prepare wheat-meal or barley-meal for baking or kneading. They will serve splendid cakes and loaves on rushes or fresh leaves." When Glaucon objects, saying "that's pretty plain fare for a feast," Socrates continues: "They will have a few luxuries. Salt, of course, and olive oil and cheese, and different kinds of vegetables from which to make various country dishes. And we must give them some dessert, figs and peas and beans, and myrtle-berries and acorns to roast at the fire as they sip their wine. *So they will lead a peaceful and healthy life, and probably die at a ripe old age,* bequeathing a similar way of life to their children."

7

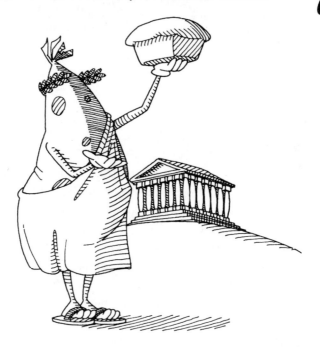

8   "There is no disease, bodily or mental, which adoption of vegetable diet and pure water has not infallibly mitigated wherever the experiment has been fairly tried."

—*Percy Bysse Shelley*

Vegetarianism helps fight impotence. Think about this: Real men don't eat meat. A high-fat, meat-based diet can curb a man's interest in sex, says Dr. A. Wayne Meikle, professor of endocrinology and metabolism at the University of Utah School of Medicine. Fatty foods, such as cheeseburgers and fried chicken, make men fat, and men with higher body fat have sunken testosterone levels, he notes. Furthermore, a

9 high-fat diet can lead to impotence. Diets high in fat clog the arteries that send blood pumping to the penis. Arterial blockages are a major source of impotence.

Vegetarians do not contribute to the suffering of cattle. Male cattle in the beef industry are routinely castrated, *almost always without anesthetics.* The two main reasons cited 10 for this painful, barbaric practice are to create a more docile, easier to handle animal, and to produce an animal that gains more weight more quickly and is thus more profitable. The castration procedure involves pinning the animal down, slitting the scrotum with a knife, exposing the testicles, and ripping them out.

11 *You will always have something to talk about.* When people learn you are a vegetarian, they will view you alternately with skepticism and curiosity. They will ask you questions about your diet, giving you an opportunity to inform and inspire. One who responded eloquently and sometimes humorously to questions about his vegetarian diet was British playwright George Bernard Shaw, who died in 1950 at the age of 94. He became a vegetarian in his early twenties, and throughout his long life he formulated a number of replies when asked about his "unconventional" diet. Most memorable was his response to one inquiring mind that he simply did not care to dine on corpses.

October will mean more than Halloween. October is designated "Vegetarian Awareness Month." There are two goals for the month:

1. To increase awareness of the many, and often surprising, environmental, economic, ethical, health, and humanitarian benefits of a vegetarian lifestyle.

2. To promote personal and planetary healing with respect for all life.

For more information, contact the sponsor: Vegetarian Awareness Network, Box 321, Knoxville, TN 37901.

12

13 *Carotene decreases the incidence of cancer.* Cancer is a major killer in North America. One of the factors that stimulates the development of cancer is a high-fat diet associated with heavy meat consumption. Vegetarians not only consume a naturally low-fat diet but also eat more of the plant foods that protect the body against cancer. One example is carotene, a chemical that the body converts into vitamin A. It is found plentifully in carrots, sweet potatoes, mangoes, winter squash, and other red/orange plant foods, such as tomatoes and cantaloupe. Carotene has been demonstrated as an effective cancer fighter.

14

Spontaneous cancer cures are linked to vegetarian diets. One of the most fascinating studies on the health benefits of a vegetarian diet comes from the University of British Columbia, Canada. There, researchers studied the dietary style of 200 cancer patients who experienced "spontaneous regressions"—unexplained cures or reductions in tumor size. Researchers discovered that 87 percent of these patients made major dietary changes, and, for the most part, that change was a switch to a vegetarian diet.

Vegetables are the food of the gods. Here is a fascinating reference to vegetarianism from the Old Testament book of Genesis (1:29): "Then God said, 'I give you every seed-bearing plant on the face of the whole earth and every tree that has fruit with seed in it. They will be yours for food.'" (New International Version). According to Richard Schwartz, author of *Judaism and Vegetarianism,* the verse means "God's original intention was that people should be vegetarian." To further back up his claim, Schwartz notes that early Biblical figures experienced remarkable longevity during the period from Adam to Noah. Adam lived 930 years; his son and grandson lived more than 900 years; Methuselah, whose name is now synonymous with old age, lived 969 years. After the great flood, when people began to eat meat for the first time, life spans dropped closer to those of our own, he observes. "We don't use that exactly as proof," Schwartz says, "but people lived the longest when they were vegetarian in the Bible."

15

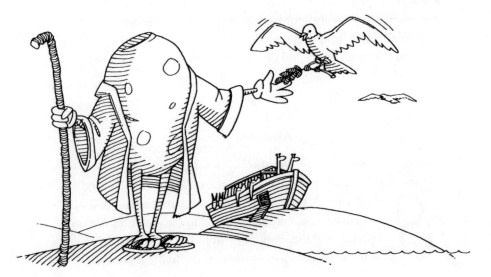

16 *Vegetarianism promotes a longer life span.* Research clearly indicates that vegetarians tend to be healthier and live longer than do omnivores. For example, a study of 27,529 adults in California was begun in 1960 and continued for twenty-one years. Meat-eaters and vegetarians were compared. The study revealed that the greater the meat consumption, the greater the death rate from all causes combined.

That study provides this interesting link to the term "vegetarian," which was first coined in the 1840s by the British Vegetarian Society and had nothing to do with vegetables. The society's founders based their name on the Latin word *vegetus,* meaning active, lively, or vigorous. At that time when the word "veget" was used in England, it described a robust, healthy person. According to the Society, the diet most conducive to a healthy, active, and vigorous life was a meatless one.

17 "There slowly grew up in me an unshakable conviction that we have no right to inflict suffering and death on another living creature unless there is some unavoidable necessity for it, and that we ought to feel what a horrible thing it is to cause suffering and death out of mere thoughtlessness."

—*Albert Schweitzer, M.D.*

18 *You can tap into the ancient wisdom of Plutarch.* Many people turn to a vegetarian diet out of concern for animals. According to the Greek philosopher Plutarch: "The obligations of law and equity reach not only to mankind; but kindness and beneficence should be extended to the creatures of every species, and these will flow from the breast of a true man, as streams that issue from the living fountain."

You will no longer be a predator. Franz Kafka, the Czech-born German writer of visionary fiction, reportedly made this remark while admiring fish in an aquarium: "Now I can look at you in peace; I don't eat you any more."

19

20

"Flesh-foods are not the best nourishment for human beings and were not the food of our primitive ancestors. There is nothing necessary or desirable for human nutrition to be found in meats or flesh-foods which is not found in and derived from vegetable products."

—*John Harvey Kellogg, M.D.*

A vegetarian diet reduces rates of skin cancer. Passing up a hamburger and reaching for something with less fat not only spares the heart and lowers your weight but may also keep your skin from developing cancer. A *New England Journal of Medicine* study reported that researchers halved the fat intake of thirty-eight people with a history of precancerous skin lesions (called *actinic keratoses*), cutting each day's percentage of calories from fat from 40 percent to 20 percent. Another thirty-eight people in the study continued their normal diets of 40-percent fat. Two years later, there were only three new lesions in the low-fat group, but there were ten among the group of thirty-eight who ate the same number of calories but didn't trim the fat. "We may have shown that a low-fat diet does the same thing that sunscreens were shown to do in an earlier study. Namely, prevent precancerous growths from arising," says the study author, John E. Wolf Jr., M.D., chair of the Department of Dermatology at Baylor College of Medicine, Houston.

21

Vegetarianism conserves the Earth's water supply. An astounding 50 percent of all water consumption is used for livestock production. It takes 2,500 gallons of water to produce one pound of meat but a mere 25 gallons to produce one pound of wheat. The rapid depletion of Earth's water supply is an increasing concern to scientists who note that water tables, such as the huge Ogalalla aquifer under the Great Plains states, are fast being depleted.

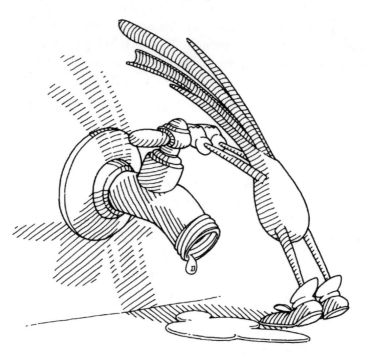

Vegetarianism is the wave of the "future." At least that was the opinion of Russian writer Leo Tolstoy, who declared: "And there are ideas of the future, of which some are approaching realization and are obliging people to change their way of life. . . . Such ideas in our world are those of freeing the laborers, of giving equality to women, of ceasing to use flesh food, and so on." With nearly 14 million vegetarian Americans, the future has arrived!

24 *Vegetarianism allows you to look at life with a touch of humor.* Surely, George Bernard Shaw, the British playwright, took delight in telling critics of his vegetarian diet: "It is nearly fifty years since I was assured by a conclave of doctors that if I did not eat meat I should die of starvation." Shaw lived a healthy and full life into his nineties as a strict vegetarian.

25 *Vegetables are the food of champions.* "Being a vegetarian has helped make me into a better all-around athlete. With the extra energy a vegetarian diet provides, I'm also enjoying a healthier and fuller lifestyle. As well as working, I carry out a rigorous training regime and participate in other sports and activities," says Roger Hughes, Welsh National Ski Champion.

Or consider these comments by Sally Eastall, a vegan (a vegetarian who does not consume eggs or dairy products) marathon runner, who has represented Great Britain in the Olympics, Commonwealth Games, and the World and European Championships: "Since becoming vegan my running has improved considerably. Vegan food is ideal—high carbohydrate, low fat and plenty of vitamins and iron. I'm proud that I run without exploiting animals in any way."

26 *Questions from others will provide you with an opportunity to tell it like it is.* "What on earth do you eat?" is a question every vegetarian receives. Here's a good response given by Nava Atlas, an illustrator and the author of *Vegetariania: A Rich Harvest of Wit, Lore, and Recipes:* "A wealth of fresh vegetables and fruits, grains, legumes, tofu, nuts, seeds, dairy products, pastas, soups, salads, good breads, and yes, the occasional dessert."

You will be following the teachings of Hinduism. Vegetarianism is a central theme of Hinduism and is formulated from the Hindu epic poem, *The Mahabharata:* "Those who desire to possess good memory, beauty, long life with perfect health, and physical, moral and spiritual strength should abstain from animal foods." Both Buddhists and Hindus believe that all life is formed and sustained through prana, or the "life force." According to this philosophy, the ideal foods are those containing life energy, such as vegetables, fruits, nuts, legumes, and grains. On the other hand, the meat of dead animals, which have lost their prana, is useless and should be avoided.

27

Vegetarianism is part of your destiny. At least that was the viewpoint of American poet and essayist Henry David Thoreau, who wrote, "It is a part of the destiny of the human, in its

28 gradual improvement, to leave off eating animals, as surely as the savage tribes have left off eating each other when they came in contact with the more civilized."

"Goodness is never one with the minds of these two: one who wields a weapon and one who feasts on a creature's flesh."

29

—*Tirukural 253 (Hindu scripture)*

30 *You will feel greater peace and serenity.* A vegetarian lifestyle opens the path to deep inner peace. Consider this observation from Chris Campbell, former U.S. Olympic medalist and now an attorney: "I don't have to kill, or have someone else kill, another living being for my support."

31 Vegetarianism promotes easier weight control. Most people know that carrying excess weight is unhealthy, yet most diets fail. A vegetarian diet will help you lose pounds and maintain normal body weight. The reason for this is that plants and grains are very low in fat and calories. Consequently, the body has a harder time producing body fat. Another reason a vegetarian diet makes weight management easier is that plant foods are high in fiber. The fiber is more filling and thus reduces the temptation to overeat.

"If you stick to a diet of high-fiber, low-fat foods—fruits, vegetables, grains, beans, egg whites, and nonfat dairy products—you can eat enough to feel satisfied and still wind up losing weight without obsessively counting calories or fat grams," says Dr. Dean Ornish, M.D., author of *Eat More, Weigh Less*.

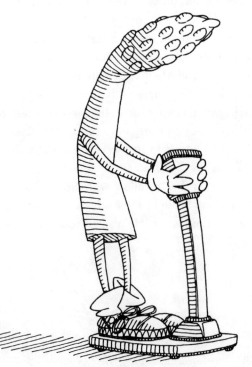

Vegetarianism lowers blood pressure. Curiosity drove Australian researcher Ian L. Rouse, M.D., to learn why Seventh-Day Adventists (they follow a vegetarian diet) tend to have lower blood pressures than the general population. Dr. Rouse decided to test sixty volunteers by switching them from a typical diet to one that was meat-free. He measured their blood pressure levels regularly. After a mere six weeks without meat, blood

32 pressures had fallen significantly. The reason for the drop is that vegetarian diets are high in polyunsaturated fat, whereas meat-based diets are high in saturated fat found in animals.

You will reverse the damage of your old diet. Current *33* research shows that dietary mistakes can be reversed by reducing the fat found in meat-based diets. Consider the experiment that Dr. James Anderson recently conducted on himself. Anderson, a medical doctor at the University of Kentucky College of Medicine began restricting calories from meat and substituting them with more grains such as oat bran. When he began his experiment, his blood cholesterol level was 285. Quickly, that count began to drop. "My blood cholesterol plummeted 110 points in five weeks, from 285 to 175," he reports. "I was the first human as far as I know to eat oat bran to lower cholesterol. The fellow who did my blood chemistry at the university lab brought the analysis over personally—he was so stunned by the results. He wanted to know what the devil I was doing."

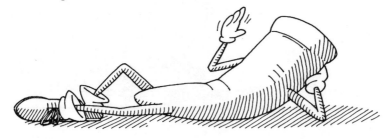

Vegetarians have better immune defenses. Eating a variety of fruits and vegetables floods the body with compounds like vitamin C and beta-carotene that boost immunity. Vegetarians consistently demonstrate that they have more vigorous immune defenses due to their diets. A recent study at the German Cancer Research Center in Heidelberg compared the blood of male vegetarians and meat-eaters. They found that vegetarians' white cells were *twice* as deadly against tumor cells as those of carnivores. That means vegetarians need only half as many white cells to do a job as meat-eaters do. In addition, the vegetarians also had much higher levels of carotene in their blood. Carotene from fruits and vegetables further strengthens the immune system.

34

35 *Your children can enter and win a vegetarian essay contest.* Children aged 18 and under are encouraged to submit a two or three page essay on topics related to vegetarianism. Essays are accepted beginning May 1st of every year, and winners are announced on September 15th of every year. Each winner receives a savings bond. For more information or to send in an essay, contact The Vegetarian Resource Group, Box 1463, Baltimore, MD 21203.

36

Your food vocabulary will improve considerably. Everyone knows about potatoes, carrots, lettuce, apples, pears, etc. However, many vegetarians can talk intelligently about *arborio* (a white Italian rice with a wide grain and creamy texture), *chipotle pepper* (a large jalapeño pepper that has been dried and smoked), *cranberry beans* (cream-colored beans with red streaks that have a nutty taste), *quinoa* (a tiny, round grain with nutty, rice-like flavor), and *red kuri* (a pumpkin-like squash with deep reddish-orange flesh and skin similar in taste to a sweet potato).

37

"A vegetarian diet is a winning diet, for health, for sport, for life. It gives me maximum energy and vitality—in fact everything I need to keep me at the peak of physical fitness and compete with the best."

—*Robert Millar, world-class professional cyclist*

38

When you want to impress friends, you can tell them you're on the "Pythagorean Diet." A contemporary of Buddha was the Greek philosopher and mathematician Pythagoras. He is best known as the originator of the Pythagorean Theorem. He is also regarded as the father of Western vegetarianism. Pythagoras, along with many other Greek philosophers, favored a natural, meatless diet. Referring to the great variety of vegetables and fruits, the mathematician noted that "the earth affords a lavish supply of riches." Vegetarianism is referred to as the "Pythagorean Diet" by many later writers, such as Ovid, Voltaire, Emerson, and Shelley.

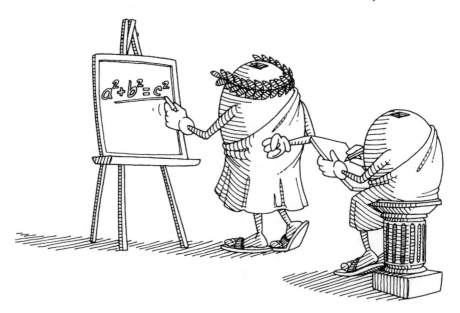

39 "If man's aspirations towards right living are serious . . . he will first abstain from animal food because . . . its use is simply immoral, as it requires the performance of an act which is contrary to moral feeling—killing; and is called forth only by greed and the desire for tasty food."

—*Leo Tolstoy*

40 *It's a weight-management diet that works.* Most weight-loss diets don't work. 97 percent of those who lose weight on traditional diets—those based on deprivation and calorie counting—gain the weight back within five years, notes Dr. Dean Ornish, director of the Preventive Medicine Research Institute in Sausalito, California. Vegetarians fare better, he says. "We studied patients who were put on a vegetarian, 10-percent fat, heart-disease-reversal diet—not a weight-loss diet. Without trying to lose weight, the average patient dropped 22 pounds the first year and kept most of the weight off for at least seven years."

41 *Vegetarians help relieve world hunger.* As a vegetarian, you will make a personal contribution to relieving world hunger by adopting an animal-free diet. Here is the logic: Land is capable of supplying food for nearly fourteen times as many people when it is used to grow food for people rather than for crops to feed animals. Cattle, for example, consume sixteen pounds of grain to yield a mere one pound of flesh. The theory promoted by those concerned about world hunger is that mass starvation could be deterred if meat-consuming societies would curtail their meat demand and use free-grazing land for the more efficient purpose of growing vegetables, grains, and fruits for human consumption.

We were designed to be vegetarians. Many scientists
note that, unlike true carnivores, humans were not
designed to eat flesh. Our intestines are much too long,
and our teeth are much too short. Even the gastric acids in our
systems say no to consuming flesh. Harvey and Marilyn
Diamond, authors of *Fit for Life,* note: "A carnivore's teeth are
long, sharp, and pointed—all of them! We have molars for
crushing and grinding. A carnivore's saliva is acid and geared to
the digestion of animal protein; it lacks ptyalin, a chemical that
digests starches. Our saliva is alkaline and contains ptyalin for
the digestion of starch. A carnivore's intestines are three times
the length of its trunk, designed for rapid expulsion of foodstuff,
which quickly rots. Our intestines are twelve times the length of
our trunks and designed to keep food in them until all nutrients
are extracted."

"If a man aspires to a righteous life, his first act of
abstinence is from injury to animals."

—*Leo Tolstoy*

It's getting easier and easier to have meat-free holidays.
While anyone can be vegetarian during most of the
year, holidays—when meals tend to be more festive—
can be a challenge for vegetarians. An increasing number of
vegetarian cookbooks are available. A good one to consider is
Vegetarian Christmas by Rose Elliot, which can be found in most
bookstores. Books by Linda McCartney (*Linda's Kitchen* and
Home Cooking) contain many festive recipes that can be used for
Christmas, Easter, baptisms, etc. Another excellent book is
*Vegetarian Celebrations: Menus for Holidays and Other Festive
Occasions* by Nava Atlas.

Meat is hazardous to health. That became dramatically evident during World War I. During the Great War, the Allies set up a blockade to prevent supplies from reaching Germany. However, Denmark was also cut off by the embargo. Lacking meat imports, Danish authorities opted to feed their grain to the people, and to do without meat. So during the war years, Danes ate cereal, potatoes, green vegetables, milk, and small amounts of butter. The result: between October 1917 and October 1918, the Danish death rate from noninfectious diseases dropped by one-third. Although other issues could be factored into that drop—more exercise and less alcohol consumption—the results proved that

 people could get along without meat, and they suggested that vegetarian diets were worth further study.

You'll stay stone-free. A vegetarian diet helps prevent kidney diseases and disorders of the urinary tract, which afflict as many as one in 100 people and will become increasingly prevalent as the population ages. A recent study of alternative and complementary therapies has established a relationship between diet and healthy renal functioning. After surveying recent medical studies, the authors of the study feel there may be a direct correlation between a diet high in animal protein and kidney stones. The reason: Animal protein increases calcium excretion in the urine, lowers urinary citrate excretion, and

46

increases uric acid content in the urine. Those three factors contribute to the formation of stones in the kidneys and urinary tract.

You would be part of a growing group of people. In 1982 there were approximately 9 million vegetarians in the country. Currently, between 12 million and 14 million Americans consider themselves vegetarians. An additional 38

47

million people say they are "careful" about how much meat they eat. Clearly, as a vegetarian you would be part of a growing group of people concerned about nutrition and health.

48

Your teen can join the Vegetarian Youth Network. This is an informal, grassroots, nonprofessional organization run entirely by and for teenagers who support compassionate, healthy, globally aware vegetarian living. The Network provides support and encouragement to vegetarian youth through various publications and communications available via phone, e-mail, U.S. mail, and the worldwide web. The Vegetarian Youth Network can be reached at: The Vegetarian Youth Network, P.O. Box 1141, New Paltz, New York, 12561. Include a stamped, self-addressed envelope for reply.

Chick peas: chock full of good things. Not only can chick peas be used to make a vegetarian "chicken soup," but this member of the bean family is winning serious respect from nutritionists. Their curiosity was raised when a study revealed that poor residents in Northern India had far lower blood cholesterol levels than higher-income residents. Suspecting that the diet of poor people, which is rich in chick peas, was a factor, researchers tested their theory. In a controlled study, chick pea consumption was promoted among wealthier families. Cholesterol levels fell dramatically—an average of 56 milligrams. Even if your cholesterol level is fine, chick peas contribute a great deal to healthy living because they provide protein, fiber, iron, and potassium, as well as substantial amounts of the B vitamins thiamin and niacin. All of those nutrients are delivered without high levels of fat or sodium.

49

50

A pumpkin becomes more than a jack-o'-lantern. Only in America is the pumpkin grown to have a face carved into it, and then to be tossed out after Halloween. But around the world, pumpkin is often eaten at every course. Not only does it have a delicious, sweet taste, but a pumpkin is high in vitamin C. Vegetarians know that a pumpkin is much more than a mere Halloween decoration. The pumpkin is a member of the winter squash family and can be used in any recipe calling for butternut or acorn squash.

"Why do you belie the earth, as if it were unable to feed and nourish you? Does it not shame you to mingle murder and blood with her beneficent fruits? Other carnivora you call savage and ferocious—lions, tigers and serpents . . . yet for them murder is the only means of sustenance! Whereas to you it is superfluous luxury and crime."

51

—*Plutarch*

Good habits will equate to good aging. Only about 30 percent **52**
of the characteristics of aging are genetically determined.
The other 70 percent are linked to lifestyle issues.
According to John Rowe, M.D., a gerontologist and director of
the MacArthur Foundation Consortium on Successful Aging,
people who lead active lives and eat healthy diets age better than
those who are sedentary and unconcerned about diet. Dr. Rowe's
observation is just another indicator of the health benefits
connected to vegetarianism.

Vegetarianism may improve your artistic work. Henry David
Thoreau also felt that his vegetarian diet improved his artistic
endeavors. In his masterpiece *Walden,* he wrote: "I believe that

53 every man who has ever been earnest to preserve
his higher or poetic facilities in the best condition
has been particularly inclined to abstain from animal
food."

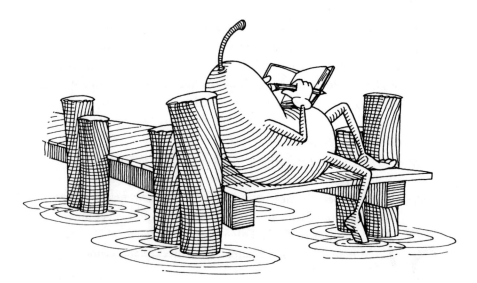

The Big Mac took a big step because of vegetarians. McDonald's, the world's largest beef purchaser, has also been influenced by vegetarians concerned about animal welfare. Recently, the chain issued a statement supporting the humane treatment of animals to all its beef and poultry suppliers. That policy statement—summarized in the company's 1993 annual report—reads: "McDonald's believes the humane treatment of animals . . . is a moral responsibility. . . . Suppliers should take all reasonable steps to assure animals raised, transported and slaughtered for McDonald's products are treated humanely." The corporation also asks suppliers to provide an annual compliance statement.

54

55

If Howard Lyman can switch, so can you. Looking at seventy people who each paid $25 for dinner and a lecture, the speaker begins: "My name is Howard Lyman, and I'm a fourth-generation farmer, rancher, feedlot operator from Montana. At one time in my life, not too long ago, I owned 7,000 head of cattle and 12,000 acres of crop and pasture to feed them. I have been personally responsible for the demise of scores of animals, and I am here tonight to tell you that the proper amount of animal products in your diet is zero," he says, linking the tip of his index finger to this thumb. Then he pauses to let the surprise of his message sink in.

During an illness that left Lyman bedridden for several months in 1979, he began reading books on environmental damage caused by agricultural pesticides. Over the course of many months, he became increasingly concerned about the waste of resources caused by the production of animal products, became a strict vegetarian, and founded the organization Voice for a Sustainable Future. Although many friends and family members vigorously disagree with Lyman, their dissent has not reduced his commitment to animal rights, environmental issues, and vegetarian living.

You'll know your beans. Because most people don't really know of too many types of beans, you can impress them with your vast knowledge of bean stock. There is the *adzuki* (which has a nutty-sweet flavor with soft texture and is often used in Asian cuisine), the *black bean* (associated with South American, Caribbean, and Mexican cooking), the *black-eyed pea* (which has a buttery smooth texture and requires no soaking), the *chick pea* (also called the *garbanzo bean*), the *cranberry bean* (with a mild, sweet, nutlike flavor), the *fava bean* (a tough-skinned bean with an earthy flavor that should be skinned before cooking), the *green bean* (commonly known as a string bean), the *kidney bean* (which has a robust flavor and a creamy texture), the *lentil* (with a light, fresh flavor, no soaking is necessary, and it cooks quickly), the *lima bean* (which has a buttery flavor and texture but should not be eaten raw), the *mung bean* (it has a sweet, soft texture and is available dried, canned, or ground into flour), the *pinto bean* (a speckled bean with earthy flavor), the *soybean* (it

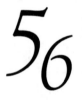

has a crisp, mild, nutlike flavor and is used to make tofu), and the *white bean* (This bean family includes the *great northern bean,* the *navy bean,* and the *small white bean.*).

Many vegetarians enjoy eating beans, which are considered by dietitians to be a true nutritional winner. Beans are rich in complex carbohydrates and fiber, and they also deliver important vitamins and minerals, such as calcium, iron, and zinc. In addition, beans are a relatively low-calorie source of protein with no cholesterol and very little fat. Vegetarians have a wide variety of recipes for their beans—everything from Boston baked beans to Cuban black bean soup, from Indian succotash to lentil soup.

Vegetarianism gives you a chance to be creative. Those who are serious vegetarians find creative ways to work around animal-based meals and celebrations. Consider Rabbi Barry Krieger of Congregation Ahavas Achim in Keene, New Hampshire. Rabbi Krieger has been a vegetarian for twenty years. Unlike most rabbis, when Rabbi Krieger holds the community-wide seder, his meal is strictly vegetarian. In a traditional seder ritual meal, several symbolic foods are presented: salt-water, representing the tears shed by the slaves, bitter herbs for the bitterness of slavery, and a shank bone, representing the lamb that would have been sacrificed to God in the Biblical days. Rabbi Krieger replaced the lamb shank bone with a boiled beet. He explains that the beet's redness is a reminder of the redness of temple sacrifices.

You reduce your risk of getting Salmonella *food poisoning.* Dr. Scott Holmberg of the U.S. Center for Disease Control says that *Salmonella* food poisoning, which comes primarily from flesh foods, strikes 2 to 4 million people each year, and one of every 1,000 dies from the illness. Most people do not realize that symptoms such as diarrhea and vomiting are often the result of contaminated animal products.

Vegetarianism can forestall baldness in men. While research in this

59

area is still evolving, Japanese dermatologists have observed that as the Japanese diet has become more westernized—that is, more laden with meat and fat—baldness has become more common, especially in younger men.

60

"I, personally, am very pessimistic about the hope that humanity's disregard for animals will end soon. I'm sometimes afraid that we are approaching an epoch where the hunting of human beings may become a sport. I personally believe that as long as human beings will go on shedding the blood of animals, there will never be any peace. There is only one little step from killing animals to creating gas chambers a la Hitler and concentration camps a la Stalin—all such deeds are done in the name of 'social justice.' There will be no justice as long as man will stand with a knife or with a gun and destroy those who are weaker than he is."

—*Isaac Bashevis Singer*

61

Eating vegetables reduces the risk of colon and stomach cancer. Cruciferous vegetables—cauliflower, cabbage, broccoli, and Brussels sprouts—appear to considerably reduce the risk of colon and stomach cancer. Norwegians, who regularly eat more of their calories in cruciferous vegetables, were found by researchers to have fewer and smaller precancerous polyps of the colon. It is worth noting that when laboratory animals eat cauliflower and then are given powerful carcinogens such as nitrosamines, they do not as readily develop cancers as those fed no cauliflower, according to research done by Dr. Lee Wattenberg at the University of Minnesota. Only 63 percent of the cauliflower-eating rats grew cancers compared with the 94 percent not given cauliflower. Scientists believe that the cauliflower contains compounds that stimulate the body's natural defense systems to neutralize carcinogens, so they don't have an opportunity to develop into cancerous tissues.

It's easier to be kosher if you are a vegetarian. Although Judaism permits the eating of flesh, there are clear guidelines about diet and restrictions on how animals are to be treated. A Torah commentator Rabbi Pinchas Peli wrote: "The laws of kashrut come to teach us that a Jew's first preference should be a vegetarian meal. If, however, one cannot control a craving for meat, it should be a kosher meat, which would serve as a reminder that the animal being eaten is a creature of God and that the death of such a creature cannot be taken lightly."

62

63 "I am astonished to think what appetite first induced man to taste of a dead carcass or what motive could suggest the notion of nourishing himself with the flesh of animals which he saw, just before, bleating, bellowing, walking, and looking about them."

—*Plutarch*

You can annoy the American National Cattlemen's Association. When former United States President Jimmy Carter gave a meatless dinner at the White House in 1977, the president of the American National Cattlemen's Association at that time responded quickly and angrily saying: "The last thing we need is the President of the United States advocating a vegetarian diet for Americans." Such an endorsement "could do great harm to the largest segment of American agriculture, the beef cattle industry," he added.

64

Like Paul McCartney, you will have more energy. The former Beatle has been a vegetarian for over twenty years. "My vegetarianism got started as a compassionate thing—and it still is—but it just happens to have environmental and health benefits," he explains. People often ask McCartney how he manages to cope with the rigors of touring now that he is in his fifties. His

65 response: "Well, I'm a vegetarian. I don't think there has ever been a night on tour when I thought, 'God, I don't have the energy to do this.'"

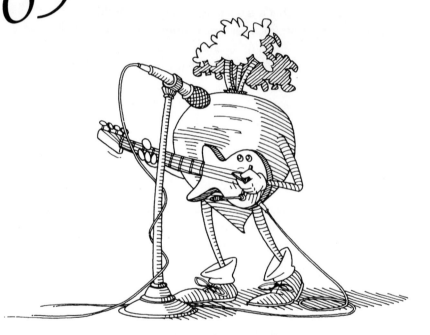

You will share a common dietary link with the ancient Sumerians. One of the earliest known civilizations was that of Sumer. Living in the southernmost part of Mesopotamia, between the Tigris and the Euphrates rivers in the area known today as Southern Iraq, Sumerians were a highly cultured, creative, and artistic people. The Sumerian language is the oldest written language in history. Sumerians were predominantly *66* vegetarian. Their diet consisted of barley cake, beans, onion, and some fish from time to time.

You won't contribute to animal cruelty. As meat consumption increases, so does cruelty to animals. Consider this piece of historical evolution: By the seventeenth century, citizens of England had become huge meat consumers. Writing in 1667, Henry Peacham noted that in England people ate more "beef and mutton in one month than all Spain, Italy and a part of France in a whole year." By 1750, England was distinguished from its European neighbors in that meat formed the centerpiece of the main daily meal. As the British appetite for meat increased, farmers and breeders responded by overfeeding animals in order to produce huge livestock. By 1800, the prize cattle paraded at the Smithfield cattle show in London were so enormous that some could barely totter around the ring. Objecting to this cruelty, some 500,000 people petitioned against the practice of producing such overgrown beasts.

Vegetarianism nourishes body, mind, and spirit— At least that is the attitude of Seventh-Day Adventists, a vegetarian Christian denomination whose members are among the healthiest people in the United States. Vegetarianism is a founding belief of Adventists. Ellen G. White, one of the founders, advised her followers to do away with meat-eating. "Vegetables, fruits, and grains should compose our diet," she said. "The eating of flesh is unnatural. Many die of disease caused wholly by meat-eating; yet, the world does not seem to be the wiser. The moral evils of a flesh diet are not less marked than are the physical ills. Flesh food is injurious to health and whatever affects the body has a corresponding effect on the mind and soul." According to Adventists, physical health, which results from a vegetarian diet, also brings greater spiritual awareness and insight.

You can intelligently answer the protein question. As soon as people learn you are eating vegetarian, they will inevitably ask: "How do you get your protein?" Most people make this simplistic assumption: Protein means meat, cheese, and eggs, while vegetables and fruit mean vitamins. When the question is asked, you have a wonderful opportunity to inform people that no one needs to rely on meat for protein. Many plant foods are high in protein—beans, grains, nuts, etc. When eaten in combinations, they provide the body with higher usable protein than do dairy or meat products. Combinations, such as rice and beans or peanut butter and bread, not only provide adequate protein, but the body utilizes and absorbs it more easily than meat protein. Most people living in North America do not need to worry about their protein intake because they normally consume plenty of food. From those meals, protein will be ingested in ways the body can use it naturally and easily.

In addition, the body maintains a "protein pool," a natural reservoir of amino acids ready and waiting to combine with whatever protein enters the body from plant sources. Although

69 dropping meat from a diet does reduce protein, the American Dietetic Association says vegetarian diets continue to meet or even exceed the recommended amount of this nutrient.

You will view violence from a different angle. Everyone is concerned about rampant crime and increasing violence in our society. Vegetarians come to understand that the senseless slaughter of animals is another form of violence in our society. The daily killing of animals reveals how little regard our society has for life. Over a lifetime, the average American citizen will eat 11 cows, 4 veal calves, 3 lambs, 43 pigs, 1,107 chickens, 45 turkeys, and 861 fish. Each American flesh-eater consumes over 250 pounds of meat and poultry each year. **70**

71

"Hold fast to vegetarianism and abstain from taking life."

—*Confucius*

It's the saintly thing to do. Yes, the famed Italian preacher, mystic, and saint famous for his love of animals—Saint Dominic—was definitely a vegetarian. "Saints seem to be overwhelmingly vegetarian," notes Jill Haak Adels, author of *The Wisdom of the Saints*. For example, Jordan of Saxony, successor to Dominic who founded the Dominican order, reported: "Never did St. Dominic, even on his journeys, eat meat or any dish cooked with meat, and he made his friars do the same." And Julia Billiart, who in the eighteenth century established the Institute of Notre Dame for the Education of Poor Children and the Training of Religious Teachers, described her vegetarian order, saying: "We have bread, salt, butter and potatoes and we are the happiest women."

72

Your rice IQ may increase. When most people think of rice, they
picture either white or brown rice. Yet there are approximately
40,000 varieties of rice grown around the world. Although it
would be impossible to sample them all, vegetarians often enjoy
more than mere white and brown rice. For example, the
thousands of different rices fall into three categories determined
by their length in relation to their width. Long-grain rices are
three to five times as long as they are wide; medium-grain rices
are at least twice as long as their widths; and short-grain rices are
anything shorter than that. You can introduce friends to these
less-known, but delicious gourmet rices: *arborio* (a medium-
grain rice used in Italian dishes), *basmati* (a long-grain rice
grown in India and Pakistan that almost doubles in length as it
cooks), *black japonica* (The bran in this medium-grain variety
dissolves during cooking, turning the water a dark purple.),
jasmine (This long-grain rice originated in Thailand but is now
grown in the United States, and unlike many rices, jasmine does
not harden when refrigerated.), *valencia* (a medium-grain rice
named for the Spanish province where it is grown, valencia adds
great flavor and texture to Spanish dishes.), and *wehani* (a

73 plump, long-grain rice grown at Lundberg Family
Farms in California that is named for its developers—
Wendell, Eldon, Homer, Albert, and Harian Lundberg).

You'll become part of a growing group of healthier people. **74**
Dean Ornish, M.D., author of the best-selling *Dr. Dean
Ornish's Program for Reversing Heart Disease,* says it
all comes down to making a healthy choice. "I grew up in Texas.
I love the taste of meat," he admits. "But frankly, I like feeling
good and being healthy much better." Like Ornish, many others
are making the switch. Statisticians report that people in
California are eating 50 pounds less of beef a year per capita.
Obviously, vegetarianism is not just a pop trend.

You benefit by enjoying foods that are more lovingly cultivated. Rice is a major food source for vegetarians. The grain has been so highly regarded by the Chinese that they traditionally greet each other with "Have you eaten your rice today?" in much the same manner that we might say "How do you do?". Among some Indonesian peoples, the belief prevails that rice contains a soul. Consequently, they treat rice in bloom the same way they would treat a pregnant woman. Loud noises are not allowed in the rice fields, lest the rice-souls be frightened, and the growing rice is fed the same foods that might be given to nourish an expectant mother.

75

76 *Your grocery list will be unique.* Carob powder, malt extract, and tofu are quite exotic for many people—the vegetarian grocery list can be unique. Once a vegetarian understands the great variety of choices available, his or her grocery list can include items such as *Hiziki seaweed, Chinese shiitake mushrooms, yuba* (bean curd strips), *buckwheat spaghetti,* and *arrowroot* (a powder used for thickening).

Your mother can say "I told you so." "Eat your vegetables" is something all children hear from their mothers. Now science is confirming your mother's belief that vegetables promote good health. In a study of 1,899 men with high blood cholesterol, those with high blood levels of carotenoids had 36-percent fewer heart attacks and deaths over thirteen years than men with low levels of carotenoids in their blood. Carotenoids are compounds that make the colorful pigments in yellow squash, green spinach, orange carrots, etc. Beta-carotene is the best-known carotenoid, but it accounts for only 25 percent of the carotenoids the blood absorbs from food. Researchers are just beginning to explore others found in vegetables.

77

78

"If slaughterhouses had glass walls, everyone would be vegetarian. We feel better about ourselves and better about animals, knowing we're not contributing to their pain."

—*Paul and Linda McCartney*

You will be walking the path of Buddha. Many Eastern nations have historically been vegetarian. Those vegetarian roots come out of their religious traditions, which have a profound respect for all life, including the lives of animals. For example, Buddha instructed: "Do not butcher the ox that plows thy field," and "Do not indulge a voracity that involves the slaughter of animals." As Buddhism spread into Japan a century later, Japanese Buddhists believed that meat-eating not only violated spiritual principles, but was physically unhealthy. They taught that eating animal flesh polluted the body for 100 days.

79

Your daily vocabulary may broaden. Most people know the word "pulse" to mean the regular beating in the arteries caused by the contractions of the heart. However, there is another meaning for the word "pulse"—the edible seeds of peas, beans, lentils, and similar plants that have pods. Pulses are among the oldest of foods consumed by human beings. Lentils, the small round seeds of a pea-like plant, have been cultivated since the earliest days of settled farming. Almost 8,000 years ago in the rich "fertile crescent" between the Tigris and Euphrates rivers (in today's Iraq and Syria) the Sumerians were growing pulses—lentils, beans, and chickpeas.

80

81 *Vegetarianism works better with your body.* Writing around 55 BC, T. Lucretius Caro made this rather modern observation: "In ancient times, lack of food gave languishing bodies to death. Now, on the contrary, it is abundance that buries them." A vegetarian diet makes weight management easy and natural while reducing the risk of various diseases associated with a high-fat, animal-based diet. Recently, R. Lee Clark, president of the American Cancer Society declared: "So far, the most likely culprit [in food-related cancer] is the high animal fat diet."

Vegetarianism is an "uplifting" way of life—That is the opinion of vegetarian and veteran actress Cloris Leachman, who says: "I'm interested in an approach to eating that is a way of life, where the road just unfolds before you and leads you into good feelings and uplifting experiences." Other vegetarian actors and actresses include Dennis Weaver, James Coburn, Paul Newman, Cicely Tyson, Gloria Swanson, and Susan St. James. Musicians include Bob Dylan, Ravi Shankar, John Denver, Chubby Checker, Gladys Knight, and the members of the band the B-52s.

82

83 "What is the good way? It is the path that reflects on how it may avoid killing any creature."

—*Tirukural 324 (Hindu scripture)*

You will always have a natural remedy. For generations, Swedish families have cited the blueberry as a remedy *84* for diarrhea and declared that this small berry can fight other infections. Swedish physicians often recommend dried blueberry soup to treat childhood diarrhea. According to Finn Sandberg, professor of pharmacology at Uppsala Biomedical Center, the typical dose is 5 to 10 grams of dried blueberries, or about one-third of an ounce. Research reveals that the blueberry is filled with high concentrations of compounds that can destroy both bacteria and viruses. In Canadian tests, crushed blueberries destroyed nearly 100 percent of polio viruses within twenty-four hours. Researchers believe that the tannins in the fruit kill the microbes. Vegetarians find many ways to enjoy blueberries: plain; with milk; in pancakes, muffins, and pies; on cereals; and as jelly spreads.

When you're tired after work, you don't have to cook. Vegetarians have it made when they've had a long, exhausting day, and they just don't feel like cooking. Unlike raw meat, which must be prepared, much of vegetarian food does not need to be cooked at all. Fruit, nuts, seeds, cheese, and fresh raw vegetables are all delicious uncooked. So, after a full day of hard labor, the vegetarian does not have to engage in *85* time-consuming meal preparation.

According to Linus Pauling, you'll have less to worry about. The two-time Nobel Prize winner, who promoted vitamin C as an effective treatment for the common cold, believed a vegetarian diet was not only healthier but also nutritionally complete for the body. "If we lived entirely on raw, fresh plant foods, as our ancestors did millions of years ago, there would be no need for concern about getting adequate amounts of the essential foods, such as vitamins," he said.

86

You will have the stamina of an ancient Roman soldier. The mighty Roman army was a nearly vegetarian one. The Romans conquered the known world with soldiers fed on bread and porridge, vegetables, a little wine, and an occasional fish. According to historian Will Durant, "The Roman army conquered the world on a vegetarian diet. Caesar's troops complained when corn ran out, and they had to eat meat."

87

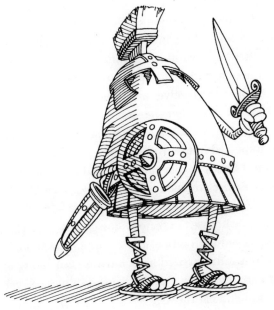

You won't have to worry about E. coli *poisoning.* Recently, many people have become sick—some violently ill—because they consumed beef products containing the E. *coli* bacteria. The fact is most flesh products can easily carry bacteria such E. *coli, Salmonella,* and others that bring about food-borne illnesses. Vegetarians don't have to worry about those. Nor do they have to fret about whether or not the cutting board was properly scrubbed and disinfected because raw meat was cut on it. In order to reduce the incidents of *Salmonella* and E. *coli* problems, poultry manufacturers are starting to rinse the poultry with chemicals in the hopes of killing off most of the bacteria. Ingesting that chemical rinse is something else a vegetarian doesn't have to worry about.

More and more scientists believe animals think and feel, so why kill and eat them? Although certain scientists continue to challenge the concept that animals are full of sense and sensitivity, the evidence is mounting against their view. Consider these examples: In Nashua, New Hampshire, a woman who depended on an oxygen tank to breathe was aided by her dog after her breathing machine stopped working. Incredibly, the dog managed to press a programmed number for 911 and bark into the receiver as it was trained to do. In Ruidoso, New Mexico, after the sudden death of a new mother, the family dog kept the woman's infant son warm for several days in an unheated house. And at a zoo in Brookfield, Illinois, a boy fell 20 feet into a gorilla enclosure and was knocked unconscious. Before anyone could come to the child's aid, a huge female silverback gorilla approached him and—instead of hurting him as witnesses expected—the gorilla tenderly cradled the boy and stayed with him to protect him. The animal understood the youth needed help. Such acts of caring and compassion are reminders that animals do think and feel. So why do we kill and eat them?

Your food preparation will rarely go wrong. Vegetarian food is not only delicious but varied, easily digested, and full of fresh delights. Menus can be extremely creative and diverse with dishes that rarely go wrong. It is the meat-eater's menu that is more likely to be limited in choices, sometimes unappetizing, and occasionally inedible. More than one person has had to chew through a leathery steak or a burned hamburger. Many people have had the experience of studying a restaurant menu, assessing their prospects for a good meal, and wishing they could go from appetizers (mushrooms in garlic, artichoke hearts) to desserts (fresh strawberry pie, cranberry pear tarts). Between the appetizer and dessert there can remain doubt about the quality of the food. Will the meat be undercooked or overcooked? Will the fish be dried out or floating in butter?

91 *"The better to see you with."* That line from *Little Red Riding Hood* is familiar to most people. However, less familiar are the results of a new study showing that vegetables protect against blindness. *The Journal of the American Medical Association* cited a study in which Harvard researchers compared 356 people who had developed a visual disorder called age-related macular degeneration (AMD) with 500 similar people who were free of the condition. With AMD, vision is blocked when tiny blood vessels grow under an area of the retina, causing scarring and hemorrhaging. Researchers concluded that people who consumed the most dark green, leafy vegetables were 43-percent less likely to develop AMD than people who consumed the least. This is yet another important rationale for vegetarianism because AMD causes vision loss in an estimated 13.1 million Americans and accounts for up to one-third of the 900,000 American cases of blindness. It makes sense for Americans to eat more dark green, leafy vegetables.

You'd fit into Mr. Rogers' Neighborhood. Of course, you may not be able to sing and play the piano like Fred Rogers, TV's "Mister Rogers," you may not have sweaters like Mr. Rogers, and you may not have your own television program, but you would be a

 vegetarian, just like Mr. Rogers. Rogers, host of the immensely popular children's program, has been a vegetarian for several decades.

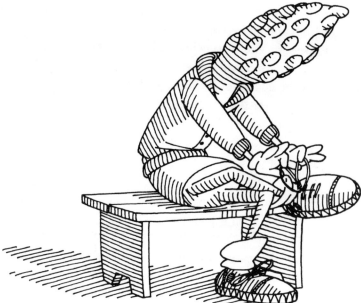

You won't contribute to the cruelty experienced by chickens. The life span of a chicken is about twenty years. However, on the factory farm, chickens are pulled from their cages in 16 to 18 months and taken to the slaughterhouse. "Redskins" is the phrase used to describe chickens who have evaded death, in spite of being hit with a powerful electrical shock, having their throats slit, and being dipped in scalding water. Those who survive this, the "redskins," are tossed, still alive, into a bin where they are later ground into feed.

94 *Vegetarianism provides variety—the spice of life.* Vegetarianism keeps you from falling into a culinary rut. There is greater variety to meals. By eliminating meat as the center of your meal, you are free to pursue new taste sensations by trying out different recipes, exotic produce, and new fruit from around the world. Vegetarianism motivates you to toss out frozen carrots and canned peas to experiment with new ways of preparing grains, vegetables, and fruits.

You will be creature-friendly. People who become vegetarians often quickly become aware of animal welfare. In being vegetarian, they don't contribute to animal cruelty. One practice that vegetarians find horrific and unnecessarily cruel is the deliberate de-beaking of breeder chickens. Although outlawed as cruel in Denmark, Holland, and Sweden, the practice is permitted in the United States. Poultry farmers commonly keep as many as a dozen hens in a cage measuring only four square feet. The crowded conditions create great stress, which causes the hens to peck each other so severely that many birds die, thus reducing egg production. Allowing chickens to run free would eliminate the pecking problem, but it would also be more expensive for poultry farmers. So they get around the issue by cutting off about half of each bird's beak with a hot blade. *95*

You will have something in common with a Nobel Prize winner. In 1978, the Nobel Prize for literature was awarded to Isaac Bashevis Singer, the American writer who was born into a Jewish family in Poland and did his writing in Yiddish. On one *96* occasion, an interviewer asked Singer whether he was a vegetarian for religious reasons or for health reasons. "It is out of consideration for the chicken," he replied.

97 *You'll have a lot of new restaurants to visit.* In cities and towns all across America, new and exciting restaurants that either are entirely vegetarian or offer a variety of vegetarian options. As a vegetarian, you will have the pleasure of discovering and enjoying many of these new restaurants. Most communities now host ethnic restaurants operated by people from Thailand, Vietnam, India, Afghanistan, the Middle East, and other primarily vegetarian cultures. There are also many books being published to help you find those restaurants, such as *Vegetarian Journal's Guide to Natural Foods Restaurants* (Garden City Park, NY: Avery Publishing Group, 1993).

98 *Sweet potatoes: bursting with beta-carotene.* One sweet potato contains more than five times the Reference Daily Intake (RDI) of beta-carotene, the precursor of vitamin A. Furthermore, they contain loads of fiber and vitamin C. Unlike white baked potatoes, which cry out for butter or sour cream, sweet potatoes have a naturally rich, moist, and sweet taste. They are delicious plain and have less than 120 calories each.

99 *You'll have more in common with Taoists.* Sixth century philosopher and founder of Taoism, Lao Tzu, experimented with plant foods, teaching his followers that overcooking vegetables destroyed their taste and nutrients. Consequently, the Taoists based their diets on raw or partially cooked vegetables. It may have been their tradition that led to the art of stir-frying. Stir-fried vegetables are barely cooked, thus retaining their color, fresh taste, and crispness. Stir-frying is an extremely popular way of cooking in many Asian countries. "We [the Chinese] eat food for its texture, the elastic or crisp effect it has on our teeth, as well for fragrance, flavor and color," noted Lin Yutang in his book *My Country and My People*. "The idea of texture is seldom understood, but a great part of the popularity of bamboo shoots is due to the fine resistance the young shoots give to our teeth."

Grapes: sweet little jewels. A vegetarian lifestyle is ideal for all those who like to sit on the sofa and snack after a hard day. Rather than reach for cookies, which are high in fat and calories but contain little nutritional benefit, eat grapes instead. These small jewels are sweet and low in calories—only 114 in a cupful! Not only will you still have the same soothing hand-to-mouth action, but grapes also contain vitamin C, potassium, and boron. Boron is a mineral that can help safeguard calcium and thereby help prevent osteoporosis.

100

You can go through the day singing musical tributes to fruits and vegetables, such as "Apples, Peaches, Pumpkin Pie," "Strawberry Fields Forever," "Yes, We Have No Bananas," "Call Any

101 Vegetable," "Glass Onion," "Lemon Tree," "Little Green Apples," "Blueberry Hill," "Tangerine," and "Don't Sit Under the Apple Tree."

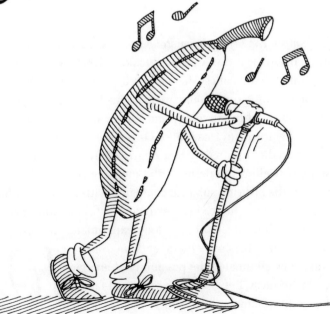

Ordering in restaurants is becoming easier for vegetarians.
Restaurants are taking notice of the increasing number of
vegetarians. In fact, the National Restaurant Association recently
commissioned a Gallup poll, which revealed that 39 percent of
those turning to vegetarianism make the switch for ethical
reasons. The same poll showed that 20 percent of all American
adults who eat out are "likely to look for a restaurant that serves
vegetarian items" and that about one-third are likely
to order vegetarian meals. Consequently, more
and more restaurants offer choices acceptable
to vegetarians.

102

103

*You can visit the many cities and towns named after
fruits and vegetables,* such as The Big Apple (New
York City); The Little Apple (Minneapolis); The
Big Potato (Moscow); Beantown (Boston); The
Oranges, New Jersey; and Lima, Ohio.

Vegetarianism can arrest rheumatoid arthritis. Give up meat, and
arthritis may fade away. A groundbreaking 1991 Norwegian study
documented that meatless diets relieved rheumatoid arthritis
symptoms in nine out of ten patients. Jens Kjeldsen-Kragh, M.D.,
of the Institute of Immunology and Rheumatology at the
National Rheumatism Hospital of Oslo reported that switching to
a vegetarian diet resulted in greater grip strength and much less
pain, joint swelling, tenderness, and morning stiffness in 90
percent of the arthritic subjects compared with those on ordinary
diets. The subjects noticed improvement within a month, and it
lasted throughout the entire yearlong experiment. According to
researchers, the diets were therapeutic not only
because they eliminated the possibility of allergic
reactions to meat, but also because animal fat
incites joint inflammation.

104

105

There seem to be only advantages and very few, if any, disadvantages to a vegetarian lifestyle.

Actually, George Bernard Shaw did cite one disadvantage to his vegetarian diet when he said: "The average longevity of a meat-eater is 63. I am on the verge of 85 and still work as hard as ever. I have lived quite long enough, and I am trying to die; but I simply cannot do it. A single beef steak would finish me, but I cannot bring myself to swallow it. I am oppressed with a dread of living forever. This is the only disadvantage to vegetarianism."

106

Beets: unbeatable vegetables. Popular with many vegetarians is the beet. One whole cup of cooked sliced beets has only 52 calories and no fat. That same cup has 3.4 grams of fiber, equivalent to one-and-a-half cups of oatmeal. Beets can be eaten raw and are delicious shredded and tossed into salads. Also, beet tops are filled with vitamin C and deliver two to five grams of fiber per cup. And beet greens, along with the greens from collard, kale, mustard, spinach, Swiss chard, and turnips, are in the cancer prevention spotlight.

107

You will be less likely to take medication you don't need. Of all antibiotics used in the United States, 55 percent are fed to livestock. Hormones, pesticides, insecticides, toxic dyes, and compounds are also routinely used on animals raised for their meat. Less than one out of every quarter million animals is tested for residues. Sick animals are treated with sulfa drugs. Hormones are regularly added to animal feed in order to accelerate growth. All of these chemicals end up in the human diet when the meat is consumed. Clearly, vegetarians avoid the danger of consuming meat laced with chemicals of all sorts.

The animal world will benefit through your vegetarianism.
According to the Farm Animal Reform Movement, 5 billion
animals live short, unhealthy, and unnatural lives of confinement
and suffering before being butchered for meat every year in the
United States. Most farm animals are not protected by law from
inhumane conditions or treatment and routinely undergo painful

108 procedures such as branding, castration,
de-beaking, suffocation, light deprivation,
and overcrowding.

Vegetarianism was the diet of Classical Greek athletes. *109*
In Classical Greece, most of the land was stripped
bare for ship construction, house building, and
charcoal. Destruction of forests caused the hillside to
be eroded, thus making poor grazing land for livestock.
Consequently, Classical Greeks did not eat much meat. In fact,
protein-rich barley was considered a most prestigious food and
was awarded to victors in the Eleusinian Games.

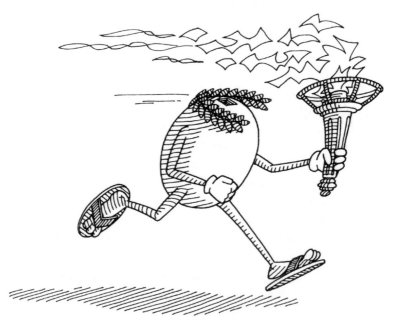

110

Quitting smoking can be easier. It's true—a vegetarian diet can make it easier to stop smoking. David Daughton, Ph.D., a nicotine researcher at the University of Nebraska Medical Center, has discovered that high-alkaline foods, such as spinach and beet greens, tend to "recirculate" nicotine in the body, thus lessening the body's need for nicotine. Foods like red meat and liver and other organ flesh tend to flush away nicotine, increasing the cravings for cigarettes. Additional foods that may make it easier to wean yourself from cigarettes include raisins, figs, dried lima beans, and almonds. Like spinach and beet greens, they all increase body alkalinity, which, in turn, recycles nicotine already present.

111

When you really think about it, eating dead flesh is unappetizing. Consider the experience of actress Candice Bergen: "I became a vegetarian when I was 22 or 23. It happened when I was in Paris and I was walking through the market district called Halles. There was just row after row of carcasses . . . and that did it for me. I could never eat meat after that."

112

Vegetarianism is heart-smart. Heart disease is a major killer in the United States and accounts for nearly half of all deaths each year. A diet high in saturated fat increases the risk of heart disease because saturated fat is turned into cholesterol, which clogs arteries. A 3-ounce hamburger contains 245 calories, and one-quarter, or 63, of those calories come from saturated fat. Researchers M. L. Burr and P. M. Sweetnam, writing in the *American Journal of Clinical Nutrition,* cite a study of 10,000 people in England who were tracked over a seven-year period. Vegetarians in the sample experienced lower death rates from heart disease than did those on a meat-based diet.

113 *Calories are not the same for vegetarians.* Here's something to think about. Vegans (the strictest vegetarians) in industrialized countries weigh an average of twenty pounds less than meat-eaters who eat the same number of calories. Thus, it is evident that calories count less for vegans than they do for meat-eaters. The explanation is actually quite simple. People who eat fat get fat. The calories consumed by meat-eaters come mainly from dietary fat found in meat. Most calories consumed by vegans come from complex carbohydrates found in grains, beans, and greens. Most meats contain no carbohydrates, and grains contain almost no fat. So vegetarians, especially vegans, have a distinct advantage when it comes to weight management.

Fresh fruits lead to a longer life. In a huge seventeen-year study of 10,771 health-conscious eaters in England, Scotland, and Wales, the people who ate fresh fruit every day, compared with average eaters who did not make eating fresh fruit a habit, had a 24-percent less chance of having a fatal heart attack, 32-percent less chance of a fatal stroke, and 21-percent less chance of dying from any cause. That information was recently reported in the *British Medical Journal.* *114*

Vegetarianism slows the aging process. Researchers are noting that one way to extend life is by reducing caloric intake. Simply stated, people who eat less tend to live longer and healthier lives. Of course, vegetarians naturally consume fewer calories by eliminating high-fat meat products. Researchers cite the example *115* of those who live in Okinawa, Japan, where calorie consumption is 30-percent below Japanese norms. The island has an unusually high percentage of centenarians.

116

The strongest animals on the planet don't eat meat. One of the main reasons cited for meat consumption is to build strength. "I need meat to keep up my strength," one carnivore might explain. Yet, the strongest animals in the world are vegetarian, including elephants, oxen, horses, mules, camels, and water buffalo. Consider the silverback gorilla. Physiologically, it resembles the human being, yet it is much, much stronger. The silverback gorilla is exclusively vegetarian, dining on fruits and other plants.

Or consider this observation from Thoreau who cited the ox as one of the world's strongest animals, but one that is strictly vegetarian: "One farmer says to me, 'You cannot live on vegetable food solely, for it furnishes nothing to make bones with,' and so he religiously devotes a part of his day to supplying his system with the raw material of bones; talking all the while he walks behind his oxen, which, with vegetable-made bones, jerk him and his lumbering plow along in spite of every obstacle."

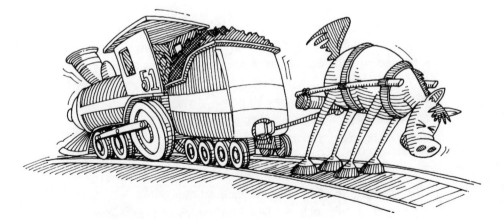

In the future, your health insurance costs may drop. Meat consumption costs Americans more than $60 *billion* annually in treatment for heart disease, obesity, cancer, and food poisoning. That figure makes meat consumption considerably more costly than the $50 *million* attributed to smoking. The insurance industry, which already provides reduced rates for lower health risk clients such as nonsmokers, is monitoring various studies identifying the health benefits of a vegetarian diet. In fact, Randall White, M.D., a professor at the Atlanta-based Emory University Medical School, believes health insurers ought to reduce premiums for vegetarians. "The data we have on the

117 general health benefits of vegetarianism would make it imperative for insurers to start rewarding people," he wrote in an editorial for *Preventive Medicine.*

You will help keep the earth green. Here are some sobering statistics: 260 million acres of American forestland have been cleared to create cropland to produce a meat-centered diet. Of those acres, 200 million could be reforested if they were no longer used for animal feed and grazing. One acre of trees per year is saved each time an individual switches to a vegetarian diet.

118

Vegetarianism lowers the risk of ovarian cancer. Eating 10 grams of saturated fat—the equivalent of one hamburger—a day may increase a woman's risk of ovarian cancer by 20 percent. However, here is the good news: Every 10 grams of vegetable fiber—the equivalent of two servings of beans—eaten daily lowers risk by almost 40 percent, reports Harvey Risch, M.D., Ph.D., associate

119 professor of epidemiology and public health at Yale University and author of a study published in the *Journal of the National Cancer Institute.* His research was based on a study of 1,000 women.

120 *The Food Pyramid—you can cut it off at the top.* Even though the United States government spent millions of dollars and several years developing the Food Guide Pyramid, you can take a vegetarian ax and cut it off at the top. Leaders of the vegetarian movement, such as Dr. Neal Barnard, president of the Washington-based Physicians Committee for Responsible Medicine and author of *Food for Life,* believe the United States food guidelines place far too much emphasis on animal products. As an example, Barnard cites the individual who, in seeking to reduce his or her cholesterol level, eats small portions of meat and removes the skin from a chicken breast. Doing that will drop cholesterol level by an average of 5 percent. "For a person with a cholesterol level of 250, that's only 12 $\frac{1}{2}$ points," Dr. Barnard notes, "nowhere near the goal of 200. But if you follow a vegetarian diet—sans all milk, eggs, and cheese—you can reduce your cholesterol level by 25 percent or more."

Dr. Barnard also feels the Food Pyramid is off-base because the latest research reveals the healthiest lifestyle is vegetarian. He notes that a diet of nothing more than grains, legumes, fruits, and vegetables can reverse the progress of coronary disease, reduce the risk of cancer and improve cancer survival, relieve arthritis, improve sexual function, reverse adult onset diabetes, ease menstrual cramps, reduce weight, and trim the grocery bill.

121 *You will have a new acronym to use—S.A.D.* Because more and more research indicates that the current meat-based diet is unhealthy, vegetarians can use a new acronym—S.A.D.—which stands for Standard American Diet. That diet is "sad" because it is loaded with fat and artery-clogging cholesterol and contains a variety of toxic chemicals.

Officials of the Russian Army know vegetarianism leads to a longer life span. Washington Post correspondent, Fred Hiatt had this interesting encounter with Russian Army officers during the Chechen conflict. While interviewing four officers, he was invited to join them for dinner, which consisted of vodka and *salo,* or cold slabs of pork fat. He declined, explaining he did not eat meat. Immediately, Viktor, one of the officers, revealed his understanding of the benefits of a vegetarian lifestyle: "You're an American. You don't smoke, you don't eat meat, and you want to live to be 90, isn't it so?"

122

You may learn something about ancient Mayan pottery. Long before Europeans descended on the Americas, the ancient Mayans and Aztec Indians developed many varieties of avocado. These peoples had high regard for the avocado, as its depiction is found on their pottery and sculptures. Eating avocados directly benefits arteries by lowering cholesterol and dilating blood vessels. Like olive oil, avocados are high in the "good" fat—monounsaturated oleic acid—which destroys cholesterol.

123

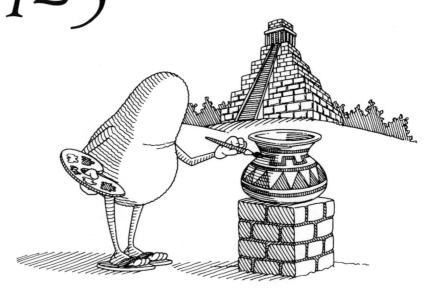

Vegetarianism is a more efficient way of sustaining life on the planet. People who study the issue of world hunger note that the planet could not be fed based on the West's meat-and-dairy-centered diet. Former United Kingdom ambassador to the United Nations Sir Crispin Tickell noted that if 35 percent of our calories came from animal products—as in most Western countries—then the world would only be able to sustain 2.5 billion people. However, if everyone became vegetarian, and the food could be equally distributed, the world could support at least 6 billion people. Thus, if everyone adopted a vegetarian diet, the combined surplus of grains and legumes would be available for the world's hungry nations.

124

Vegetarians help preserve the earth's delicate ecosystem. For more than a century, private ranchers have grazed their livestock on 270 million acres of public lands, an area equal in size to all fourteen eastern seaboard states plus Missouri. Until recently, no one really knew what impact grazing had upon endangered wildlife. Now, a study by the National Wildlife Federation (NWF), a conservation group in Washington, DC, shows that cattle grazing has contributed to the decline of at least 346 fish and wildlife species that are either on the government's endangered list or on the verge of being extinct. The endangered species are diverse and include the Apache trout, the peninsular bighorn sheep, and the western sage grouse. According to study author John Horning, "native ecosystems across the West are unraveling," as a result of cattle grazing. Grazing cattle wreak this ecological havoc in many ways: by beating out native wildlife for limited food; by trampling streamside habitats, as well as burrows, nests, and plants that provide protective cover for wildlife; by introducing and transmitting disease; and by fouling water with fecal matter. Obviously, if more people adopted a vegetarian lifestyle, this danger to the ecosystem would decrease dramatically.

125

What you eat has a lot to do with whether or not you develop stomach cancer. The truth of that statement is best expressed by Isadore Rosenfeld, M.D., in his book *Doctor, What Should I Eat?* Dr. Rosenfeld states: "Its [cases of stomach cancer] relatively low incidence and continuing decline in this country may reflect the fact that we are eating more fresh fruit and vegetables than ever before. In Japan, stomach cancer causes more deaths than all other malignancies combined and is almost six times more common than it is in the United States, presumably because of all the pickled, salted, barbecued, and smoked foods the Japanese eat. The best way to beat stomach cancer is to avoid or cut down on all of the above and eat lots of fresh fruits and vegetables that are rich in vitamins C and A."

126

127 "A dead cow or sheep lying in a pasture is recognized as carrion. The same sort of a carcass dressed and hung up in a butcher's stall passes as food!"

—*John Harvey Kellogg, M.D.*

You will be less likely to suffer from diverticulitis. Adding more fruit to your diet could protect you from a common disorder of the digestive system called *diverticular disease,* which affects a third of all Americans over age 45. When researchers from Harvard University and Brigham and Women's hospital tracked the health of nearly 48,000 men for four years, they found that diverticular disease was 42-percent less likely to occur among high-fiber eaters than among men whose diets had little fiber. Fiber from fruits and vegetables, rather than from cereals and grains, seemed responsible for the protective benefits.

128

More mighty magnesium enters your body. Health **129**
experts note that a diet rich in magnesium has
powerful therapeutic benefits. Magnesium has
the following effects on the body:

- It reduces blood pressure.

- It lowers heart attack risk.

- It increases energy level. ATP, the body's energy molecule,
  can't help the body produce energy without magnesium,
  which is an essential element in almost every energy process
  within the body.

- It prevents tooth decay. Magnesium helps prevent the need
  for extensive dental work by helping calcium bind to tooth
  enamel.

The best sources of magnesium are nuts, legumes, whole
grain cereals and breads, dark green vegetables, and soy foods—
all important staples of a vegetarian diet.

130 *Being a vegetarian helps fight bacterial and
viral infections.* Eating plenty of spinach,
carrots, and other fruits and vegetables
rich in beta-carotene boosts immune
defenses against bacterial and viral infections, as well as cancer.
In one study of sixty men and women (average age 56), beta-
carotene increased the percentage of specific infection-fighting
immune cells, says Ronald R. Watson, Ph.D., at the University
of Arizona, Tucson. The more beta-carotene, the greater the
increase in protective immune cells. Vegetarians often consume
a diet high in carotene foods naturally because they often
consume such foods as spinach, kale, sweet potatoes, pumpkin,
squash, tomatoes, and carrots in abundance.

You can have the body that is right for you. As a physician, Dr. Neal Barnard is very concerned about people who adopt "milkshake" diets in order to lose weight and obtain the body type that they are comfortable with. "Those things [the diets] are tantamount to torture, and they are dangerous," he says. The cycle of dieting and gaining leads to problems such as bulimia and anorexia, he notes. In his opinion, "vegan diets are simple compared to most weight control diets. You can eat as much as you want, and the weight will come off naturally. It's not a diet. It's a lifestyle change." And it's a change Barnard says people will

131 enjoy. "What I see is people getting into a body that is right for them. They don't have to resolve themselves to a life of pain, or an extra 30 or 40 pounds."

You can advise people how to do it. If you are already a vegetarian, others will view you as the "expert" and will solicit your advice to guide them. Here are some tips you can pass along:

132

- Do it gradually.
- Try new foods and experiment.
- Be patient.
- Subscribe to a vegetarian magazine for motivation and new recipes.
- Read and learn about vegetarianism.
- Study nutrition.
- Ignore the critics.
- Enjoy yourself and have fun.
- Buy some new cookbooks.
- Be strong.
- Stick with it.

A vegetarian diet deters diabetes. Scientists have noted that diabetes is rare among Africans, Asians, and Polynesians, who eat primarily starches, vegetables, and fruits. But when the same people switch over to a meat-based American diet, diabetes increases dramatically. Beans and other legumes are especially effective in controlling diabetes. In several studies, type I diabetics, those who need daily insulin shots, cut their insulin needs by 38 percent when they consumed one cup of cooked beans per day. Those with type II diabetes (adult onset diabetes), who do not produce enough insulin on their own, virtually eliminated the need for any injections of insulin. Researchers believe that beans produce slow rises in blood sugar so that the body needs to release much less insulin to keep the glucose under control.

133

"What is virtuous conduct? It is never destroying life, for killing leads to every other sin."

—*Tirukural 312, 321 (Hindu scripture)*

You'll be intimately involved with phytochemicals. People who consume large amounts of plant foods are flooding their bodies with *phytonutrients*—healing compounds found in plants. Many studies reveal that phytonutrients help prevent a variety of diseases. For example, *lycopene,* found in tomatoes and red grapefruit, protects against cell damage. *Chorogenic acid,* found in green peppers, strawberries, and tomatoes, blocks production of cancer-causing nitrosamines. Another example is *genistein,* found in soybeans and tofu. It helps prevent small tumors from growing. These and hundreds of other phytonutrients begin working in the body when plant foods are consumed.

135

136

The Detroit News *food editor praised vegetarian diets.* Robin Mather, food editor at the *Detroit News* recently applauded vegetarian diets when she wrote: "We who eat meat should remember that it's not the healthiest choice." In that column, Mather cited the "staggering" medical statistics that point to the benefits of vegetarianism for long life and a healthy body. She also said, "Life can be good without meat at the center of the plate."

137

"To my mind the life of a lamb is no less precious than that of a human being. I should be unwilling to take the life of a lamb for the sake of the human body. I hold that the more helpless a creature, the more entitled it is to protection by man from the cruelty of man."

—*Mahatma Gandhi*

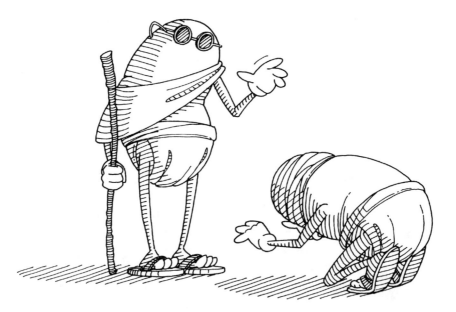

Take a lesson from the Bible: When you dine at the king's table, you're asking for trouble. Interestingly, the ancient Biblical book of Daniel provides a quick lesson in nutrition and health. In the very first chapter of Daniel, you can read a report that may be the first nutritional study ever recorded. There we learn that the king so valued Daniel and his three companions because of their wisdom that he assigned a servant to them, instructing him to feed the four men his diet, made up of rich foods (fit for a king) and wine. However, Daniel insisted on eating only vegetables, grains, and water. The servant was concerned the king would be angry if Daniel and his friends became ill as a result of their vegetarian diet, so Daniel suggested a ten-day experiment against a control group. Here was his request: "Give us nothing but vegetables to eat and water to drink. Then compare our appearance with that of the young men who eat the royal food." (Daniel 1:12-13, New International Version).

Eating only vegetarian food and drinking fresh water, Daniel looked healthier and better nourished than the men who ate the king's diet. Somehow, Daniel knew that the fatty foods set on the royal table were unhealthy. Rather than subject his body and mind to that disease-inducing diet, he ate nutritious vegetables and grains and drank pure water. By using the men who ate the king's food as a control group and himself and his companions as the experimental group, he showed the benefits of a nutritious, low-fat diet.

Vegetarian food is delicious! A nationwide Gallup poll reveals that 88 percent of those surveyed about vegetarian food indicate that health consideration is a main reason for their diet choice. However, an amazing 86 percent of those surveyed also cited taste preferences as a reason for choosing vegetarianism. The bottom line: Vegetarian food is delicious.

The hamburger is becoming a symbol of global ecological destruction and environmental degradation. That is the view of Dr. Michael W. Fox, a vice president of the Humane Society of the United States and director of the Center for Respect of Life and Environment in Washington, DC. He notes that meat, a major export from South America and Australia, has led to the

140 destruction of forests for the purpose of opening up land for raising cattle. Such forest reduction accelerates the spread of deserts and contributes to the greenhouse effect.

Vegetarianism is hot! The National Restaurant Association (the other NRA) believes that vegetarianism is hot and on the rise. In fact, the NRA has recommended that its 150,000 member restaurants feature meatless main dishes and even add whole vegetarian sections to their menus. That *141* advisory was prompted by a nationwide Gallup poll, revealing that one out of every five restaurant-goers actively seeks out eateries serving vegetarian food, and that one out of every three diners will order non-meat dishes, when available.

142 *Aging: No one lives forever, but it's worth a try.* Today's nutritional wisdom declares that lowering the fat, cutting the meat, and piling on the veggies is good for your weight and your health. Now there's even more good news. A major study published in the *British Medical Journal* followed about 6,000 vegetarians and 5,000 equally healthy meat-eaters (the mean age was 39) for twelve years. Here is what the researchers found: The meatless group was about 40-percent less likely to die from cancer and was also about 20 percent less likely to die for any reason during the study period. While no one lives forever, vegetarians definitely live longer and healthier lives.

There's something "fishy" about fish. Some people who attempt to follow a vegetarian diet continue to include fish in their diets. However, fish "reflect the pollution of the waters they come from," writes Sharon Yntema, author of *Vegetarian Pregnancy: The Definitive Nutritional Guide to Having a Healthy Baby.* "Swordfish, marlin, and bluefish are particularly dangerous, and any fish from the Great Lakes or the Hudson River should be completely

143 avoided during pregnancy (and in general). Freshwater carp, wild catfish, lake trout, mackerel, striped bass, and whitefish are likely to contain high levels of PCBs and also should not be eaten."

The U.S. military is anticipating more vegetarians. Although not yet a common meal item, shelf-stable *144* vegetarian field rations have been developed by the U.S. military. Obviously, military officials have spotted the trend among the civilian population and anticipate that more and more soldiers will request vegetarian meals.

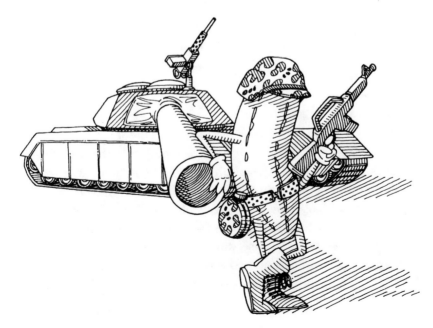

145 *Vegetarianism is the diet of a marathon ice skater.* David Phillips, a vegetarian and world-class skating marathoner from Long Island, New York, is one of the country's few long-distance skaters. Phillips is also a vegetarian. Recently, he participated in the grueling 200K marathon held in the Arctic circle town of Rovaniemi, Finland. "I didn't go to win: I just wanted to survive," says Phillips, who battled brutal arctic gusts, while avoiding skater-swallowing crevices for eight hours and twenty minutes. To get in shape for such an exhausting race, Phillips either cycles 250 miles or in-line skates 100 miles a week all year long. Just as important as building leg muscles is building up energy stores to power those muscles for so many hours. Phillips loads up on carbohydrate-rich pastas and potatoes and other vegetables right up to race time. During a race, he carries energy bars and bottles of a glucose-based energy drink. He also consumes vast amounts of the "nearly frozen" bananas that race officials hand off to skaters.

"Animals are my friends, and I don't eat my friends." *146*
                    —*George Bernard Shaw*

147 *The USDA is concerned about the health hazards of meat consumption.* Following the 1993 E. coli outbreak, the United States Department of Agriculture (USDA) spent more than $500 million to hire 200 new meat inspectors. However, outbreaks of poisoning from E. coli, *Salmonella,* and other food-borne illnesses continue. Furthermore, the USDA conservatively estimates that 15 percent of meat and poultry carcasses are contaminated with disease-causing bacteria.

Protect your joints—eat more pasta. Most people know that loading up on carbohydrates before a competition can improve endurance. Now experts identify another benefit to eating pastas, breads, potatoes, and other foods high in carbohydrates before a major physical activity: It may reduce injury. Becky Zimerman, R.D., a staff dietitian for the National Institute for Fitness and Sports in Indianapolis, says: "It's not just fuel—your muscles need those stored carbohydrates to make repairs, too." She notes that when the muscles run out of carbohydrate calories, they become weaker, and that can result in an injury. A diet without meat means you will naturally consume more carbohydrates and thereby provide yourself with this additional benefit.

148

Dr. pepper can help you heal. Sweet red peppers often cost two times more than green ones, but they might be worth it. Red bell peppers contain nine times as much beta-carotene, a precursor

149

of vitamin A, as green peppers do. Vitamin A is a disease-fighter known to speed the healing of wounds. Also, red peppers have more than double the vitamin C of their green cousins.

150

You can further worry the meat industry. With more and more people eating more and more vegetarian fare, the meat industry has become very concerned. Recently, the beef industry mounted a counter-attack against the country's move toward vegetarianism, in which they declare beef as "real food for real people." And pork producers are promoting their product as "the other white meat" to interest people who avoid red meat in favor of chicken and trukey, white meats perceived as healthier choices than beef. In spite of more aggressive meat advertising, vegetarianism continues to gain more and more adherents.

"It had something to do with eating things that had a face."

—*Fred Rogers, on why he became a vegetarian.*

151

152

Planes, trains, and automobiles will give you more pleasure. Many people find it hard to get excited about taking a trip because they experience motion sickness. This is where vegetarians have an advantage. Researchers are demonstrating that high-fat meals can increase motion sickness. In a recent study, volunteers were placed in a rotating drum after eating. Some consumed a low-fat meal, while others ate mainly high-fat food. Those who ate the high-fat meal were far more likely to experience nausea than those who ate the low-fat meal. The conclusion that researchers made: Avoid fatty foods before airplane flights or car or train trips if you are prone to motion sickness. Of course, the easiest and most natural way to eat low-fat regularly is by following a vegetarian diet.

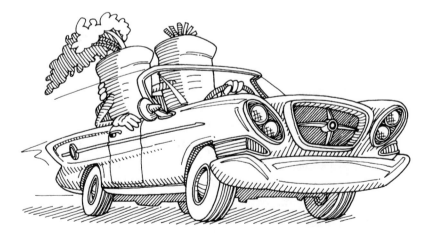

You can celebrate World Vegetarian Day. October 1st is designated World Vegetarian Day. Sponsored by the North American Vegetarian Society (Box 72, Dolgeville, NY 13329), the day celebrates vegetarianism's benefits to humans, animals, and the planet.

153

Garlic contains anti-aging properties. Another plant food with many benefits is garlic. And it does more than merely add extra zest to a pasta sauce. Preliminary research from Denmark strongly suggests that garlic has anti-aging properties as well. When researchers there added garlic to human skin cell cultures they were growing in a lab, the cells survived longer and even kept a "youthful" appearance longer than cells grown with standard nutrients. The same researchers also found that garlic blocked the growth of cancerous cells in the test tube. Of course, further research will be necessary before these findings can be directly applied to humans, but these early studies are just another argument in favor of a plant-based diet.

154

You will have less risk of disc degeneration. A meat-based diet, high in fat, can do more than expand the belly. It may also hurt the lower back. In a recent study of the arteries of eighty-six average-weight men, the greater the amounts of deposits of fatty plaque there were, the greater the degeneration of spinal discs. According to the researchers, diminished blood supply, caused by the clogged arteries, affects discs, muscles, nerve roots, and other structures in the lower spine. The positive note for vegetarians is this: A low-fat diet reduces the risk of such disc degeneration. And for those who switch from a meat-based diet to a plant-based one, their switch to a low-fat diet may minimize further disc degeneration.

155

156 *Vegetarianism is a weapon against disease.* Yes, this theme recurs throughout the book, but consider this additional information. One comprehensive, groundbreaking study conducted by researchers at Cornell University over a seven-year period studied over 6,000 Chinese people. Because the Chinese eat few animal products, researchers were especially interested in noting the relationship between diet and the risk of developing certain disease. Here's what they found:

- The average Chinese adult, whose fiber intake is three times greater than that of the average American, is two to three times less likely to develop colon cancer than an American.

- Although the rural Chinese consume more calories than most Americans do, they are much thinner. This is because their plant-based diet means that only 15 percent of their calories come from fat, whereas Americans routinely consume 40 percent of their calories as fat.

- The cholesterol levels of the Chinese are almost half those of typical Americans. That, in turn, means heart disease is much rarer in China than in America.

Clearly, vegetarianism is a weapon against many diseases.

Small changes produce big gains. Even a switch to a *157* partial vegetarian diet rewards people with better health. Consider Robert Land, M.D., and medical director of the Osteoporosis Diagnostic and Treatment Center in New Haven, Connecticut. Although he eats an occasional piece of chicken and some seafood, he experienced dramatic improvement from several health conditions once he changed his diet. "I eat no red meat at all and practically no dairy products," he says. "Once I adopted that diet, my allergies cleared up by about 90 percent and my asthma by 95 percent. My colitis problems are practically nonexistent."

158

"I resolved to abstain from flesh meat, and at the end of a year the habit of abstinence was not only easy, but delightful."

—*Seneca*

George Foreman recommends vegetarianism for natural weight loss and management. World heavyweight champion boxer, George Foreman, has always had a problem with weight management. He has learned to cut back and even eliminate meat products and other high-fat foods in order to maintain his weight at a healthy level. For others struggling to lose weight, Foreman advises eating more fiber found in whole grains, fruits, and

159

vegetables. "When my weight really gives me a hard time, I go strictly vegetarian for two weeks to a month. The weight always disappears," he notes.

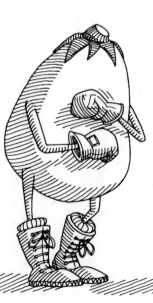
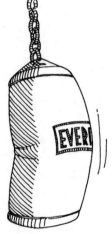

Vegetarianism often leads to other healthier lifestyle changes. When they asked 150 vegetarians and an equal number of nonvegetarians the same questions about their lifestyles, researchers at the University of Texas, Austin made many important discoveries.

Nonvegetarians had been hospitalized during the previous five years more than twice as many times as had vegetarians. Twice as many nonvegetarians reported having taken prescription medications as had vegetarians. Almost three times as many vegetarians abstained from alcohol as had nonvegetarians. Only half as many vegetarians smoked as did nonvegetarians. Almost thrice as many vegetarians practiced meditation on a regular basis as did nonvegetarians. Vegetarians overwhelmingly believed they were healthier than did the nonvegetarians. Vegetarians went out socially with friends and entertained friends at home more often than did meat-eaters. More vegetarians had actively lobbied for legislation within the previous two years than did nonvegetarians. Of those who had lobbied for legislation, more vegetarians were concerned with environmental and energy issues than were nonvegetarians.

Vegetarian food hits the slopes. Many vegetarians have avoided taking up skiing for fear of starving to death. For years, most restaurants at ski slopes provided the basic burgers, fries, and milkshakes. This is finally changing as more and more ski slopes offer vegetarian fare. Many restaurants in major ski towns—in Colorado, Pennsylvania, Vermont, California, and Canada—are featuring a variety of meatless dishes. Their "new" choices include vegetarian lasagna, pizza, sandwiches, soups, and diverse salad bars. This is just another sign that vegetarianism is growing in acceptance and popularity.

New vegetarians report positive first impressions. "Did you feel any different when you first became a vegetarian?" is a question most vegetarians hear. Interestingly, there is a common theme that runs throughout answers to that question. Most vegetarians report that they feel more energetic, healthier, "lighter," and less prone to depression. Other vegetarians tell of more dramatic changes that they've experienced, relating how switching from a meat-based diet to a plant-based one resulted in the disappearance or diminishment of various conditions, including heartburn, arthritis, and even cancer.

162

Vegetarians have speedier metabolisms. It seems vegetarians have an advantage over nonvegetarians in the inevitable slowing of metabolism and the resulting weight gain that occurs with aging. A recent study indicates that vegetarians have an 11-percent higher resting metabolic rate (RMR) than do nonvegetarians. This is very good news because a reduced RMR places a person at

163 increased risk of becoming overweight and developing weight-related health problems, such as heart disease, stroke, and diabetes.

Vegetarian diets protect against osteoporosis. Cornell University researchers also discovered that osteoporosis, the bone-thinning disease, is far less common in China. This, in spite of the fact that the Chinese eat few dairy products and consume only half as much calcium as do Americans. Researchers noted that the health benefits enjoyed by the Chinese are related to their diet. An impressive 75 percent of their calories come from complex carbohydrates—rice, grains, and vegetables. So it seems that complex carbohydrates are another valuable weapon in the fight against osteoporosis.

164

165

Livestock production is wasteful and inefficient. Some vegetarians refer to meat as "second-hand vegetables" and note that feeding grains to animals is a circuitous way of producing food for people. It is quite wasteful and inefficient. In the United States, livestock eat 145 million tons of grain and soy per year but produce only 21 million tons of animal products. Surely, no car owner would appreciate buying 145 gallons of gas but only being allowed to use 21 gallons.

You would help reduce the federal deficit. The water to produce livestock comes primarily from irrigation projects and government subsidies, which are paid for with tax dollars. Much of these tax dollars could be saved if more people switched from

166

a meat-based diet to a vegetarian one. It is estimated that if the meat industry absorbed those costs, meat would cost as much as $30 per pound.

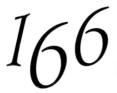

Vegetarians have double protection against many forms of cancer. Studies dating back to the 1960s on Seventh-Day Adventists, most of whom follow vegetarian diets, consistently demonstrate that the group has a significantly lower death rate from many forms of cancer, including lung and breast cancers. Initially, cancer researchers believed that the low amounts of fat in their diets was the key factor in this good health. However, new research indicates that vegetarians have double protection against many forms of cancer. Researchers are learning that there is something more to vegetarians' general good health than merely avoiding animal fat. "Probably the most striking result of our work is that no matter what cancer site we examine, there seems to be a very strong protective association with the consumption of fruits and vegetables," says Paul K. Mills, Ph.D., who has studied the Adventist diet and lifestyle for many years.

Alice Giles is a vegetarian. "Who is Alice Giles?" you are probably wondering. Giles is a world-class harpist and has been a vegetarian for over a decade. Giles was introduced to vegetarianism by a friend while she was studying in Cleveland. She tried it initially for whatever health benefits there could be: "If it's healthy, I'll try it," she says of her attitude at the time. Soon after adopting the diet, she did indeed feel better. "I had been very sick because of all the stress of the first year at school," she recalls. "I had throat infections constantly. But after that first year, I wasn't sick at all." In fact, Giles believes her energy is higher because she is a vegetarian. When she needs even more energy for performances or recording sessions, she fine-tunes her vegetarian diet to an even more "pure" state. "I give up sugar and sweets and caffeine," she explains. "This helps me keep going." When she is in between performances, Giles indulges in an occasional cup of tea or piece of chocolate.

You can tell people the difference between a fruit and a vegetable. A fruit is the ripened ovary of a plant. This would include such "vegetables" **169** as tomatoes, squashes, avocados, and peppers. A vegetable is a plant cultivated for its edible parts, such as its roots, flowers, leaves, or stems.

You'll have a better bladder. When Dr. Paul K. Mills, Ph.D., studied cancer among Seventh-Day Adventists over an eight-year period, he discovered a startling association between meat **170** consumption and bladder cancer: "A twofold increase in bladder cancer risk was associated with frequent meat consumption," he noted. "Meat consumption turned out to be very risk enhancing" for future bladder cancer problems.

You'll have one less worry in life. Vegetarians have reduced problems with constipation. Defined as infrequent and difficult bowel movements, constipation is experienced by 23 percent of women and 9 percent of men, studies reveal. It is caused by many things, including a blockage in the digestive system, lack of exercise, and a diet deficient in fiber. Americans annually spend an estimated $750 million on laxatives. However, laxatives are not a long-term solution to constipation. In fact, laxatives can worsen the problem because they can be habit-forming. Once the body begins to rely on laxatives to prompt bowel movements, the body's natural mechanisms are weakened and can shut down. But constipation is seldom, if ever, a problem among vegetarians because they naturally **171** consume a high-fiber diet. Also, the fiber tends to make stools softer and bulkier, so they pass more easily and frequently.

There is evidence that animal foods can lead to hearing loss. In populations where there is heavy meat consumption, hearing levels tend to be low. Russians living in Moscow, where the average diet is rich in animal foods, for example, have substantially lower hearing levels than those living in the Georgian Republic, where the average diet is rich in plant foods. In a study comparing over 300 Muscovites with the same number of Georgians, hearing in the Georgians over age forty was significantly better than the hearing in the Mucovites over the age of forty. Also, hearing was excellent for Georgians over 100 years old. Researchers were quick to note that noise trauma associated with urban living did not explain the differences. The hearing levels of the Georgian factory workers were better than those of the Moscow factory and clerical workers together, although the Moscow clerical workers were exposed to lower levels of noise and should have had better hearing. The key difference between the two groups is diet.

172

You'd be following the diet of Matthew, the disciple. Christians who are thinking about a vegetarian lifestyle may be interested in the fact that Matthew, a disciple of Jesus, was reported to be a strict vegetarian. That information comes from Clement of Alexandria, a prominent leader of the early Christian church. Denouncing meat-eaters as "gluttons," he reminded his hearers that **173** "the apostle Matthew partook of seeds and nuts and vegetables without flesh."

174 *Even if you're a strict vegan, you will get enough protein.* A major concern expressed about vegetarianism is protein. However, even the strictest vegetarians—vegans, who eat no meat, fish, chicken, dairy, or egg products—get more than enough protein from their diets. Dr. Patricia K. Johnston, associate dean of Loma Linda University's School of Public Health has studied the protein question. She says that even vegans usually get 50 or 60 grams of protein per day, well beyond the federal government's RDA (Recommended Dietary Allowance) of .36 grams per pound of body weight. That works out to approximately 43 grams per day for a 120-pound woman.

175 *Vegetarianism is the diet to beat back fatigue.* Increased energy continues to rank high on the list of positive changes experienced by those who switch to a vegetarian diet. "Nearly one out of every three vegetarians reports an enhanced level of energy, stamina, and endurance, making this the most commonly mentioned health-related benefit," write Paul R. Amato, Ph.D., and Sonia A. Partridge in their book *The New Vegetarians: Promoting Health and Protecting Life.* "Many people who notice an improvement in energy are involved in sports or athletics. Not surprisingly, they find that giving up meat is associated with better performance."

Vegetarians take the "Golden Rule" one step further. Jesus taught his followers: "So in everything, do to others what you would have them do to you." (Matthew 7:12, New International Version). While agreeing wholeheartedly with that teaching, vegetarians extend it to the animal world as well. Thomas Hardy wrote: "The establishment of the common origin of all species logically involves a readjustment of altruistic morals, by

176 enlarging the application of what has been called the Golden Rule from the area of mere mankind to that of the whole animal kingdom."

Say good-bye to gallstones. Many people suffer with lumps of solid material, usually cholesterol, that form in the gallbladder. These lumps are called gallstones. Vegetarians have greater protection from gallstones than do nonvegetarians. In one study, Fiona Pixley and her colleagues from Oxford University compared 632 women who ate meat with 130 women who were vegetarians. They found that the meat-eaters' risk of developing gallstones was twice that of the vegetarians. Pixley also noted that Africans, who have a traditional diet high in fiber, rarely develop gallstones. **177**

You'll still be able to eat "cheese." Many who switch to a vegetarian diet also try to limit (or even eliminate) dairy products because they tend to be high in fat. That includes cheese, which frustrates some vegetarians who love Italian food. However, more and more cheese substitute products are being developed that can be added to Italian dishes. Many of them are soy-based. One company even

178 makes a Parmesan alternative that is dairy-free, casein-free, and lactose-free so that lovers of Italian food can once again adorn their spaghetti, mostaccioli, and lasagna with a little "cheese."

179

"I do not regard flesh-food as necessary for us at any stage and under any clime."

—*Mahatma Gandhi*.

An apple a day can keep the cardiologist away. A five-year study of 805 Dutch men found that those with the highest consumption of flavonoids (natural antioxidants) were about half as likely to die from heart attacks as those with the lowest consumption. That was reported in the medical journal *Lancet*. The flavonoids in the men's diets came mainly from tea, apples, and onions. Many vegetarians naturally consume more flavonoids than nonvegetarians and thus have lower incidences of heart problems.

180

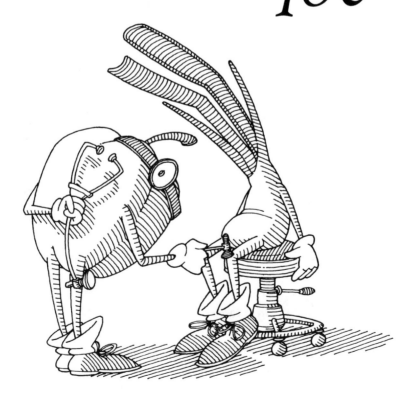

Broccoli: Stalk trouble before it starts. A team of researchers at Johns Hopkins University School of Medicine in Baltimore made the front page of the *New York Times* with their discovery: A potent compound called *sulforaphane,* which is found in broccoli and other cruciferous vegetables, causes cells to speed up their production of enzymes known to protect against cancer-causing chemicals. "Although the story is not yet complete," says researcher Paul Talalay, M.D., a molecular pharmacologist who heads a program at Johns Hopkins to develop strategies for protection against cancer, "our prediction is that sulforaphane will block tumor formation in animals and presumably man." This study is just another example of the fact that many staples of the vegetarian diet contain compounds that have cancer-protecting properties.

181

Vegetarianism is the diet that heals. Research done by heart disease specialist Dean Ornish, M.D., demonstrates that when it comes to heart disease, a vegetarian diet heals the heart. Dr. Ornish placed twenty-eight patients with hardening of the arteries (atherosclerosis) in an experimental group comparing them with twenty people with the same condition who received the traditional medical treatment for atherosclerosis. The experimental group was asked to eat a low-fat (less than 10-percent calories from fat) vegetarian diet. At the conclusion of the one-year experiment, even Dr. Ornish was surprised by the results. At the beginning of the study, both groups had about the same severity of heart disease. This was not true after twelve months.

Eighty-two percent of the patients who followed the low-fat vegetarian diet experienced a regression of their clogged arteries. Dr. Ornish was amazed and impressed to note that

182

their arteries were less clogged than before the study began, while the group treated with traditional medicine ended up with arteries that were more clogged.

183   Vegetarianism can repair damaged hearts. In the same study by Dr. Ornish as mentioned in entry #182, patients in the vegetarian group reported a 91-percent reduction in the frequency of chest pains (angina), a 42-percent reduction in the duration of angina, and a 28-percent reduction in the severity of their angina.

In contrast, the group treated traditionally continued a downward trend in terms of heart health. They experienced a 165-percent rise in the frequency of angina, a 95-percent rise in its duration, and a 39-percent rise in the angina severity.

184   You will feel good when the weather is bad. Many people suffer from SAD (Seasonal Affective Disorder), a type of depression caused by diminishing sunlight in the winter months. One remedy for SAD is to follow a vegetarian diet because it's low in fat. Researchers believe that high-fat meals fill the bloodstream with fat, making less oxygen available to the brain. Sleepiness and low energy result, further contributing to the feelings of lethargy and depression. SAD researchers note that carbohydrates can lift one's mood. Specialists in SAD relief often recommend eating less fat by consuming more carbohydrates in traditional vegetarian fare such as breads, cereals, pastas, and grains, as well as fruits and vegetables.

185   Your concept of love will be expanded. Most vegetarians develop a higher awareness of animal welfare. That includes a feeling of greater love and sensitivity toward the various creatures that share the planet with humans. In her book *Black Beauty,* Anna Sewell makes this insightful statement: "There is no religion without love, and people may talk as much as they like about their religion, but if it does not teach them to be good and kind to beasts as well as man, it is all a sham."

King Lear's Spears may improve your love life. Asparagus, often referred to as "King Lear's Spears," was first gathered by the Greeks. They discovered it growing wild on the shores of the Eastern Mediterranean. By the year 200 BC, the Romans were cultivating it. Asparagus came to America with the first European settlers. Many consider asparagus to be an aphrodisiac, and it is cited in love poetry by the early Greeks. Chinese and East Indian literature also refer to asparagus as a food that can improve one's love life. Madame Jeanne Antoinette Pompadour, mistress to King Louis XV of France, served asparagus often, drizzling it with a lemon and butter sauce. And sexologist Van de Velde included asparagus as one of the best all-around "love foods." In addition to whatever sexual power asparagus may have, it is definitely rich in potassium, phosphorus, and calcium. Also, six medium spears contain a mere 20 calories.

186

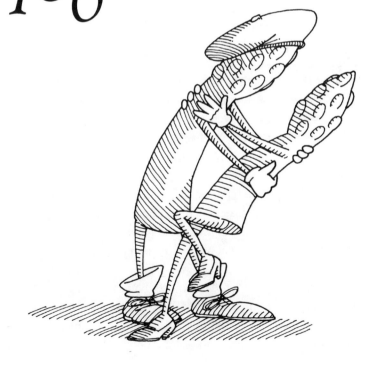

Your immune system will be stronger. Our immune systems protect us from hostile elements in our environment. When our immune systems are healthy, we can come in contact with germs and not get infections, with allergens and not have allergic reactions, and with carcinogens and not get cancer. While there are many ways to protect the immune system, diet plays an important role. Andrew Weil, M.D., author of *Natural Health, Natural Medicine,* suggests reducing "foods of animal origin." "Meat, poultry, and dairy products often carry residues of antibiotics and steroid hormones that can weaken immunity." In the place of flesh foods, Dr. Weil recommends precisely what vegetarians consume routinely: "A low-protein, high-carbohydrate diet with plenty of fruits, vegetables, and fiber is good for immunity, as well as general health." *187*

188 For women, there's relief from PMS. Although there is not firm evidence that a vegetarian diet is the answer to every woman's premenstrual syndrome (PMS) troubles, some women do experience relief when switching to a diet of plants and fruits. Judith Wurtman, Ph.D., a researcher at the Massachusetts Institute of Technology, believes a high-carbohydrate, low-protein diet can reduce or eliminate some of the more prevalent symptoms. Working with nineteen subjects who lived at her lab for three to five days before their periods, Wurtman fed the subjects only a bowl of corn flakes moistened with nondairy creamer for the duration of the experiment. "It worked like Valium," she reported. Women who were morose and sluggish, suddenly became alert and happier, Wurtman added. Dr. Wurtman's belief is that carbohydrates (contained in the corn flakes) raise the level of a brain chemical called *serotonin,* which is a mood and sleep regulator. Wurtman gave the women corn flakes without milk because the protein in the milk would curtail serotonin production. The bottom line is that a diet low in fat and protein, but high in complex carbohydrates (fruits, vegetables, and whole grains) can bring relief for PMS.

You'll be in step with the Framingham Heart Study. **189** Here's a quote worth thinking about: "Of all the diets we have out there to choose from, the vegetarian [diet] is obviously the best. Everything else [is] a compromise." That declaration comes from William P. Castelli, M.D., director of the famed Framingham Heart Study and lecturer in preventive medicine and clinical epidemiology at the Harvard Medical School.

190 *Getting started is easy.* If the idea of being a vegetarian appeals to you, but you feel overwhelmed by the thought of changing your diet overnight, start by eating a few meatless meals each week. Then, gradually increase your amounts of vegetarian meals consumed until meat is completely absent from your diet. Also helpful is visiting a bookstore or library to select some new vegetarian cookbooks.

Veggie meals are winners. Yet another sign that vegetarian eating is growing in popularity is the fact that Linda McCartney's line of Home Style Cooking Meatless Entrees was recently selected as one of the year's six best new food products. That decision was made by the editors of *Food Processing* magazine. Because there were 8,000 possibilities to choose from, the competition was intense. Here are the criteria by which the winners were chosen. "We wanted those [products] that were the most intriguing," not just variations on an already popular product, explains field editor Jim Wagner. The products also had to be successful in seizing sizable market share and capturing the hearts of shoppers. McCartney's product fit the bill. According **191** to *Food Processing,* more than 100 million of the frozen meals have been sold in the United Kingdom, capturing nearly 25 percent of Britain's $152 million meatless-meal market.

192

Tomatoes: the joy of dieting. A tantalizing thought about the tomato—tomatoes are so low in calories that you could eat two a day for an entire summer and never gain an ounce. One whole cup of tomatoes has just 35 calories but lots of potassium, vitamin C, and beta-carotene. Here's an amazing story for you to consider. Graham A. Colditz, M.D., and associates at Harvard Medical School interviewed more than 1,000 people about their diets, then tracked their health for five years. As astonishing as it may seem, the cancer rate was lowest among those who ate tomatoes or strawberries every week. It's possible that this is just a scientific coincidence, but the nutrient profile of the tomato— rich in vitamin C, beta-carotene, and fiber—fits right in with the cancer prevention recommendations made by the National Cancer Institute. So, enjoy the tomato. If you want to enhance color, flavor, taste, and texture of soups, salads, sauces, and sautés, just add tomatoes.

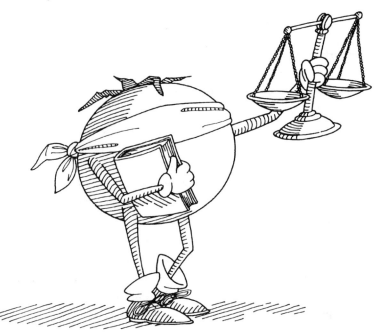

Speaking of tomatoes, here's an interesting historical note. The argument over whether the tomato is a fruit or a vegetable was actually settled by the U.S. Supreme Court in 1893. This is how the high court came to its decision. According to the Tariff Act of 1883, fruits could be imported duty-free, but vegetables could not. In 1886, one importer argued that since tomatoes were botanically fruits, he should be able to bring them in duty-free. A legal battle raged all the way to the Supreme Court. After hearing the arguments, the Court determined that, although tomatoes are a fruit of the vine, as are squashes, beans, and the like, they, as "all those vegetables . . . are usually served at dinner . . . and not, like fruits generally, as a dessert." Thus, tomatoes were pronounced to be vegetables by law.

193

"I know, in my soul, that to eat a creature who is raised to be eaten, and who never has a chance to be a real being is unhealthy. It's like . . . you're just eating misery. You're eating a bitter life."

—*Alice Walker*

194

You will be in greater control of your health. By eating a vegetarian diet, you exercise a natural and greater control over your general health. Study after study documents the direct health benefit of a plant-based diet. Most recently, the *New England Journal of Medicine* published a study that showed that cholesterol levels can be reduced with the use of soy products. Subjects who increased tofu and other soybean products while reducing animal proteins cut their total blood cholesterol levels by an average of 9.3 percent. Not only were the results of eating vegetarian fare positive, but results came quickly as well. The subjects saw results within six weeks to three months after making the switch.

Fabulous fiber leads to a good gut. In spite of widespread
advertising urging people to eat more fiber and less meat, the
average American consumes only 14.8 grams of fiber per day.
And that's not enough. The daily recommended amount is 20
to 35 grams of fiber. Those who eat that amount cut down their
risk of diverticular disease, that painful bowel condition, by one
half. Out of 47,888 men studied for four years, 385 developed
diverticuli, tiny pouches in weak intestinal walls, which
announce themselves through cramps, a bloated feeling, or
bleeding. When researchers looked at what the men habitually
ate, they saw that men eating the most fiber (32 grams or more
daily) had a 42-percent lower chance of getting diverticular
disease than did men who ate the least (13 grams). Men eating
beef, pork, or lamb as a main dish more than two to four times
a week had more than three times the risk of acquiring the
disease, compared with men who ate such meals less than once a
month. Most of the benefit came to people who consumed large

195 amounts of fruits and vegetables. A vegetarian
diet, which is naturally high in fiber, virtually
eliminates the problem of diverticular disease.

You can keep Father Time on hold. Not only is a diet
made up of fruits and veggies the key for long-lasting
health, researchers have also discovered that it has *196*
the ability to reduce and delay illnesses and diseases connected
to the aging process. One example of a fruit with such
capabilities is watermelon. It is rich in a substance called
glutathione—an antioxidant compound whose multitalents
include knocking out cancer-causing invaders and strengthening
immunity. Our bodies manufacture glutathione, but as we age,
our levels drop. Scientists are not sure why that happens. So,
rather than resent the fact that a watermelon is taking up the
entire refrigerator, look at it as your secret anti-aging medicine.

You can eat like a weight lifter. Although Andreas
Cahling is a 210-pound professional bodybuilder
from California who has won the championship
title Mr. International, when he sits down to eat, his

197

meals consist of such items as lentil loaf, mashed potatoes,
oatmeal, fruits, beans, vegetables, grains, whole wheat pasta,
green salads, brown rice, soy milk, and vegetable juice.
Adhering to a similar diet is actress, stuntwoman, and
bodybuilder Spice Williams. The clearly muscled 145-pound
woman is capable of squatting 315 pounds. Even though the
training of these bodybuilders is vigorous and physically
demanding, meat is conspicuously absent from all of their
meals. Cahling and Williams, along with an increasing number
of professional and amateur bodybuilders, are vegetarians who
have discovered that a vegetarian lifestyle provides them with
an extra edge in their training.

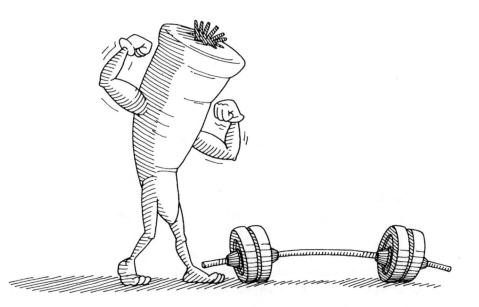

If you're Jewish, you can enjoy meat-free holy days. Several organizations have responded to requests from Jewish vegetarians for recipes for meatless meals, especially at festive, holy times of the year. The Vegetarian Resource Group (Box 1463, Baltimore, MD 21203) has compiled a list of meat-free Passover recipes. For a vegetarian seder, contact "Haggadah for the Liberated Lamb" in Hebrew and English from Micah Publications (255 Humphrey St., Marblehead, MA. 01945).

198

A meat-based diet cannot feed the world. A hungry planet of over 5 billion people cannot continue to be fed with an inefficient and wasteful meat-based agriculture. An increasing number of scientists are talking about the need for a sustainable agriculture for the planet. Sustainable agriculture is essentially one that produces fruits and vegetables for human consumption. A meat-based agriculture is not sustainable because non-renewable resources—land, topsoil, water, and fossil fuels—are squandered to raise food primarily for farm animals and not for people.

199

The desire for flesh-foods is artificially conditioned. If you look closely at the habits of children, you will realize that the desire for meat is not natural. Young children find animals to be a source of comfort and tenderness, as is made evident by the many stuffed animals children enjoy sleeping and playing with. Most children are reluctant to eat meat when they find out exactly what it is. Thus, author Ashley Montague raises this question in his book *Of Man, Animals and Morals:* "Do we have the right to rear animals in order to kill them so that we may feed appetites in which we have been artificially conditioned from childhood?"

200

201

You will be the beneficiary of a big payoff. Consider this insight from Dr. Dean Ornish. In the introduction to his 1994 paperback edition of the best-seller *Eat More, Weigh Less*, Dr. Ornish writes an apologia for the title. He says what he truly wanted to name his book was *How to Help Prevent Heart Disease, Obesity, Stroke, Breast Cancer, Prostate Cancer, Osteoporosis, Diabetes, Hypertension and Lots of Other Illnesses*, but he was afraid "you might not read it." For years now, Dr. Ornish, a heart specialist, has been promoting the value of a low-fat, vegetarian diet. He appeals to people to change their lives through diet and by nurturing their spiritual and emotional selves. The payoff is a longer, healthier life, which will allow you to eat and play with your grandchildren, rather than being fed through a tube in a nursing home.

202

"To abstain from the flesh of animals is to foster and to encourage innocence."
—*Seneca*

203

As a vegetarian you will think more about the sanctity of all life—human and animal. Even though many begin a vegetarian diet primarily for the improvement of health, their eating habits often quickly lead them to look differently at animals. The following observation by the Right Reverend John Austin Baker, Bishop of Salisbury, England is one that most vegetarians would agree with: "The saddest of all fates, surely, is to have lost that sense of the holiness of life altogether, that we commit the blasphemy of bringing thousands of lives to a cruel and terrifying death, or of making those lives a living death—and feel nothing."

You can be Irish and vegetarian on St. Patrick's Day.
It's true, holidays can be tough for vegetarians. 2O4
Historically, most people celebrate special days
and occasions by bringing on the meat. There is turkey at
Thanksgiving, ham at Easter, and corned beef on St. Patrick's
Day. However, vegetarians are becoming increasingly creative at
trading in the old meat-based foods for new and unusual
sensations for holidays. More and more vegetarian cookbooks
offer alternative dishes for traditional holidays. So on St.
Patrick's Day you can be Irish and vegetarian. For example, one
recipe from *Vegetarian Times* magazine calls for vegetarian
"corned beef" and cabbage. The meal includes cabbage, onions,
potatoes, and carrots, along with various spices, canola oil,
horseradish, and white wine vinegar. The end result is a
delicious meal with far fewer calories and fat than a traditional
corned beef meal.

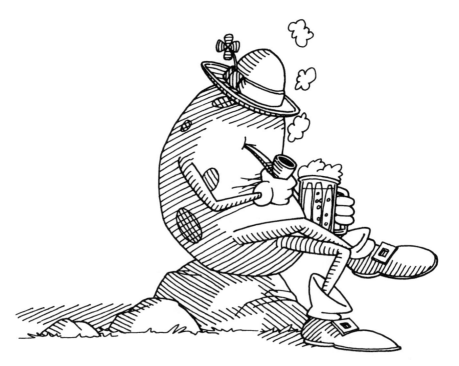

205

Factory farming is hazardous to your health. In order to raise the largest animals possible in the shortest period of time, new methods are employed on the factory farms. Often they can be hazardous to human health. For example:

- 40 to 50 percent of the antibiotics used in this country each year are administered without medical supervision to factory-farmed animals. In addition, growth hormones, arsenic appetite stimulants, sulfa drugs, nitrofurans, coloring agents, fungicides, insecticides, and recycled wastes are routinely added to animal feed.
- In a 1990 test of milk distributed in the New York City area, 80 percent of the milk tested contained tetracycline.
- Chicken parts, including intestines, are recycled into chicken feed. Industry experts believe this may be a major factor in the now rampant epidemic of *Salmonella* poisoning.
- The Enteric Diseases Branch of the National Centers for Disease Control estimates that between 400,000 and 4,000,000 cases of *Salmonella* may occur each year. A report on infectious disease published by the Carter Center in Atlanta, Georgia, estimates that at least 500 people die unnecessarily each year from *Salmonella* poisoning. Also, studies reveal that one out of every three chickens sold in the supermarket is infected with live *Salmonella* bacteria.

206

You'll help keep the earth cleaner. Factory farm animals produce 250,000 pounds of excrement each second. Much of that winds up, untreated, in our streams, lakes, and groundwater. Obviously, if everyone (or at least a sizable portion of the population) became a vegetarian, this problem of waste would be reduced considerably.

You can help save the rain forests. The tropical rain forests of Central and South America, home to half of all the living species on earth, are being decimated to produce hamburger meat for fast-food restaurants because of the high demand for meat.

207 According to authorities, this loss of rain forest is responsible for most of the 1,000 species extinctions each year.

You will not be involved in the "slaughter of the innocents." The foundation of a meat-based diet is the suffering and destruction of millions **208** of nonhumans. Even though animals are nonhumans, they exhibit "human" emotions, such as fear, depression, and compassion. For example, a chimpanzee may die of grief if something happens to his or her mother. Whales are reluctant to leave an injured member of their pod, often at the risk of their own safety. A pig, confined for months in a stall as it is fattened for consumption, becomes chronically depressed or engages in unnatural aggressive behavior. Animals can be viewed as "innocents" who are slaughtered to meet the artificially conditioned dietary "needs" of humans.

209 *You get back more than you give up.* That's the opinion of nutritional consultant Suzanne Havala. "I relish my vegetarian lifestyle, because I love the way it makes me feel. I have not been sick in years—no colds (not even a sniffle), no flu—I stay sickeningly healthy. I feel good, I have boundless energy, I never have indigestion (even when I pig out), and I control my weight effortlessly." Suzanne also says that feeding her body a low-fat, vegetarian diet is like giving it "super premium, unleaded fuel." It helps her keep in top shape and maintain a hectic schedule and fast pace of life.

210 *14 carrot gold.* Carrots, along with other deep yellow and orange vegetables, are packed with beta-carotene, an antioxidant that is converted into vitamin A in the body. Like all antioxidants, beta-carotene aids in preventing disease. In a study published in *The American Journal of Clinical Nutrition,* people with low intakes of carotenes were found to be at a greater risk of developing lung cancer than those with carotene-rich diets. Other research demonstrates a link between carotene-rich diets and lowered incidences of breast and bladder cancers. If that isn't enough to convert you into a carrot-munching fiend, consider the fact that researchers say by adding a mere two carrots a day to your diet, you can reduce cholesterol by as much as 20 percent. That, in turn, helps lessen the threat of heart disease. Furthermore, a large carrot has just 31 calories.

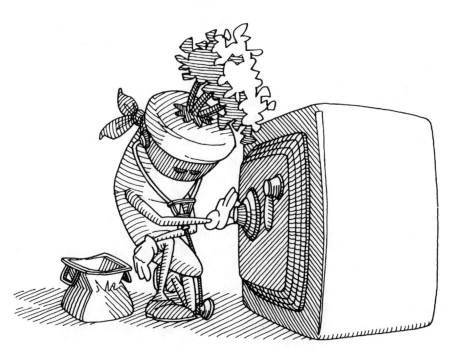

Vegetarianism is the silver lining in a dark future. Ecologists predict that the dinner table of the future will look like this: grains, beans, veggies, and virtually no meat. Although Americans may not voluntarily become vegetarian, they may be forced involuntarily to adopt such a diet. According to a report by the Washington, DC-based Carrying Capacity Network (CCN)—a non-profit group that researches the connections between economics, population growth, and environmental degradation—Americans will be pushed to a primarily vegetarian diet by the year 2050 due to a burgeoning population and dwindling tracts of cropland. "In the next sixty years [the U.S.] population will double, while at the same time 120 million acres of farmland will be lost," declares David Pimentel, Ph.D., professor of agricultural sciences at Cornell University and co-author of the CCN report. "Under those conditions, you're not going to be able to grow enough grain to feed the huge numbers of livestock that will be needed to satisfy the meat appetite of 520 million Americans." Although that is a dark view of the future, there is this 211 silver lining, says Dr. Pimentel—the plant-based diet of the future will be better healthwise.

212 *Because animals suffer.* In the 1600s, philosopher René Descartes declared, "I think, therefore I am." Because animals didn't appear to think, many who were influenced by Descartes, viewed animals as mere automatons, incapable of pain, suffering, pleasure, or thought. Thus, animals could be treated any way that a human being considered appropriate—either kindly or cruelly. Vegetarians are more comfortable with the concern for the treatment of animals espoused by philosopher Jeremy Bentham. Writing in the 1700s, he rebelled against common attitudes toward animals by declaring: "The question is not, 'can they reason?' nor 'can they talk?' but, 'can they suffer?'." His insight endures as a moral compass for many vegetarians and those involved in today's animal rights movement.

213

A more balanced diet leads to a more balanced environment. A vegetarian diet is not only healthy for you, but it is also good for the planet because a meatless diet conserves the earth's natural resources. For example:

- Agriculture is the leading cause of water pollution in the United States. Most of the pollution is due to livestock manure.
- Fifty times more fossil fuels are needed to produce a meat-centered diet than for a vegetarian diet.
- Forests throughout the world are being destroyed to make room for cattle grazing. Between 1960 and 1985 alone, 40 percent of all Central American rain forests were destroyed to create pasture for beef cattle.
- An acre of trees is spared each year by each individual who switches to a meatless diet.
- The production of a pound of beef requires 2,500 gallons of water. More than half of all water used in the United States goes to livestock production.
- It takes less water to feed a vegetarian for a year than it does to feed a meat-eater for a month.

214

Your high-fiber diet will mean fewer doctor visits. As least a dozen studies have linked diets high in fiber with a lowered risk of colon cancer. While scientists are not exactly certain why this is true, they believe it has something to do with the fact that the fiber moves foods through the digestive tract more quickly. "It decreases transit time, and therefore, anything harmful is in contact with the bowel for a shorter period of time," says Gladys Block, Ph.D., professor of public health and nutrition at the University of California, Berkeley.

215 *Some vegetarians rocket to success.* Leslie Alexander, owner of the champion Houston Rockets basketball team is a vegetarian who is enthusiastic about the many benefits of his diet. "I love tomatoes," he says, and he adds pasta and potatoes to his list of vegetarian favorites. Alexander, a vegetarian for several years, adopted his meatless diet for health reasons and because his wife, Nanci, taught him about the suffering that factory farm animals endure. He has made dramatic changes. For example, bacon and eggs, once among his favorite foods, have been completely eliminated from his diet. Vegetarian meals are always available on the plane when he flies with the Rockets. Alexander's influence can be seen among many of the Rockets players who are also learning the benefits of greens and grains.

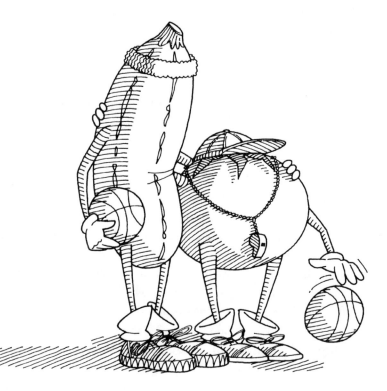

You can have a cleaner conscience. Not only is a vegetarian diet better for *you*, but it indirectly helps feed other people, especially those in poorer nations who are on the edge of starvation. Here are some amazing statistics:

- One acre of pasture produces about 165 pounds of beef, *but the same acre can produce 20,000 pounds of potatoes.*
- If Americans reduced their meat consumption by only 10 percent, there would be 12 million more tons of grain to feed humans, enough to feed each of the 60 million people who starve to death each year.
- It takes 16 pounds of grain to produce a pound of beef. The American livestock population consumes enough grain and soybeans each year to feed more than five times the entire American population—1.3 billion people.

Because Old MacDonald's farm is a myth. Many women and men become vegetarians out of concern for animals and their treatment. The children's storybook pictures of farm life where animals frolic freely under the care of a benevolent farmer is gone. Old MacDonald's farm has been replaced by what is called "factory farming." That phrase is applied to the new style of farming that has emerged over the last fifty years. The factory farm is a place where the objective is to turn out high volumes of a standardized product at minimal cost per unit. Every year, nearly 5 billion animals are slaughtered in the United States alone. Most of these animals are raised in intensive, high-volume, mechanized factory farms. Although animals thrive on affection, they receive no compassion or affection on a factory farm. Factory farmers simply have too many animals and have neither the time nor the desire to get to know them.

According to editors of the Harvard Health Letter, *you should veg out!* The latest nutritional buzz phrase at this time is "functional foods." According to editors of the *Harvard Health Letter,* that phrase refers to "foods with ingredients thought to prevent disease." The article cites growing scientific evidence that eating certain vegetables helps to protect you from various cancers. At least 200 studies from around the world show that a plant-rich diet lowers the risk for many kinds of tumors. Twenty-three studies reveal that a diet high in grains and vegetables cuts the risk of colon cancer by 40 percent. Another study shows that women who eat few vegetables have a 25-percent higher risk of getting breast cancer. So intriguing are these studies that scientists at the University of Illinois are studying phytochemicals and other components of plant foods that seem to interfere with the cancer process—slowing, stopping, or even reversing it. **218**

219 "If you have men who will exclude any of God's creatures from the shelter of compassion and pity, you will have men who will deal likewise with their fellow men."

—*St. Francis of Assisi*

You'll be ahead of your time. The issue of animal rights is coming up more and more in our society. Many vegetarians have always felt compassion for other creatures. Here is a pithy, **220** insightful comment from British novelist Brigid Brophy: "To us it seems incredible that the Greek philosophers should have scanned so deeply into right and wrong and yet never noticed the immorality of slavery. Perhaps 3,000 years from now it will seem equally incredible that we do not notice the immorality of our own oppression of animals."

Ben Franklin recommended a vegetarian diet as a thrifty way to live. During the eighteenth century, Benjamin Franklin experimented with vegetarianism, giving up meat at age sixteen. His primary appeal was the thriftiness of the diet. In fact, he convinced his employer, a printer whom he described as a "great glutton," to consider a vegetarian diet. "He agreed to try the practice if I would keep him company," Franklin wrote. "I did so and we held it for three months. We had our victuals dress'd, and brought to us regularly by a woman in the neighborhood, who had from me a list of forty dishes, to be prepar'd for us at different times, in all which there was neither fish, flesh, or fowl, and the whim suited me the better at this time from the cheapness of it, not costing us above eighteen pence sterling per week."

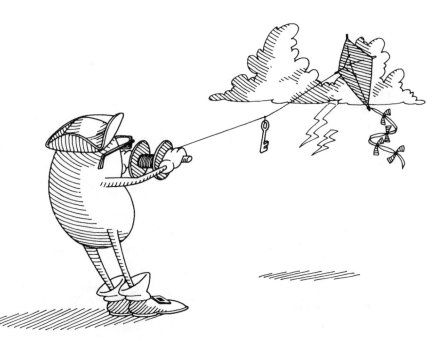

You can tell people why you don't feel at "home on the range."
When people learn you are a vegetarian or are considering
becoming one, many will say: "Meat has always been part of the
human diet, so why not continue to eat it?" Setting aside the
issue of animal rights, there are three compelling responses:

1. Modern meats may be up to seven times as fat as meat eaten
   in earlier times. Modern meats are quite different from the
   meats of 100 years ago, when genetic engineering and
   scientifically selective breeding for specialized, meatier body
   types were unknown.

2. Modern meats are additionally unhealthy because they
   are often laced with residues from the drugs and chemical
   additives the animals have ingested during the course of
   their lives. The full consequences for humans of this long-
   term exposure through their food is not yet known.

3. In the industrialized wealthy nations of the world, more
   meat is being consumed than ever before
   in history. Thus, comparing today's meat
   consumption to that of prehistoric and
   ancient civilizations is improper.

223 *The joy of soy.* Soy brings good news for
women. A single serving of tofu each day
may lower a woman's risk of developing breast
cancer, says Kenneth Setchell, Ph.D., director of clinical mass
spectrometry at Children's Hospital Medical Center in
Cincinnati. Tofu, rich in protein, is made from the soybean. For
several years, Dr. Setchell has been researching the soy/breast
cancer connection. Although he points out that a major clinical
study must yet be undertaken before the direct link between soy
intake and decreased risk for breast cancer is proven, he believes
"all the evidence is pointing in the right direction."

224 *There is a "divine-like" aspect to a vegetarian lifestyle.* In the Age of Reason, Thomas Paine wrote: "The moral duty of man consists of imitating the moral goodness and beneficence of God manifested in the creation toward all His creatures. Everything of persecution and revenge between man and man, and everything of cruelty to animals, is a violation of moral duty."

225 *You will not unwittingly be part of agricide.* A meat-based diet not only has an impact on personal health, but it also adversely affects the environment. As more and more people turn to meatless eating, a deadly trend may be reversed. In his book *Agricide,* Dr. Michael W. Fox notes: "It must be apparent that we cannot go on as we have been. We are killing the earth, killing the animals, killing ourselves—this is the true meaning of Agricide."

226 *You can use the month of June to educate and inform others about vegetarianism.* June is National Fresh Fruit and Vegetable Month. It's a good time to remind people of the abundance, variety, good taste, good value, and importance to good health of fresh fruits and vegetables. You can receive more information by contacting the sponsor: United Fresh Fruit and Vegetable Association, 727 N. Washington St. Alexandria, VA 22314.

You'll know more about the "honey" in "honeymoon." Honey, a favorite among many vegetarians, may be good for romance. Honey has been placed high on the list of aphrodisiac foods by ancient cultures, especially Greece and Rome. In fact, the word "honeymoon" was dubbed in ancient Europe, where newlyweds were encouraged to drink a mixture of honey and wine in order to heighten their amatory stamina. Today, honey's good reputation stems from the fact that it's one of the most easily digested and absorbed energy sources. Also, honey is high in B vitamins and protein, "which are vital for healthy sex," notes Cynthia Mervis Watson, M.D., author of *Love Potions*.

227

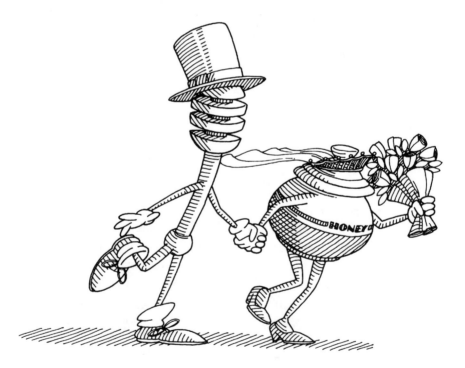

Lung-lasting care. It is known that nonsmokers have lower rates of lung cancer than do smokers. New research indicates that when it comes to lung cancer, what you eat may be as important as what you breathe. One of the largest studies of foods and lung cancers in nonsmokers to date notes that fruits and vegetables should be a main course in the fight against the disease. Researchers studied the eating habits of 413 nonsmokers with lung cancer and 413 healthy nonsmokers and found that those who ate more than two and one-half servings of raw fruits and vegetables a day had a 60-percent lower risk of lung cancer than people who ate one serving or less of those foods each day. "In terms of reducing your risk of lung cancer, our results would suggest that raw-fruit-and-vegetable consumption may be as important, if not more important, than avoiding passive smoking," said study leader Susan Taylor Mayne, Ph.D., director of the cancer prevention and control research program at the Yale Cancer Center.

228

229

"As long as man continues to be the ruthless destroyer of lower living beings, he will never know health or peace. For as long as men massacre animals, they will kill each other. Indeed, he who sows the seed of murder and pain cannot reap joy and love."

—*Pythagoras*

230

You will expand upon the meaning of compassion. By avoiding flesh foods, vegetarians expand what it means to live compassionately on the planet. Dr. Albert Schweitzer observed: "Compassion . . . can only attain its full breadth and depth if it embraces all living creatures and does not limit itself to mankind."

Consumption of fruits and vegetables cuts stroke risk. A recently published study revealed that an increase of three servings per day of fruits and vegetables was associated with a decrease in risk of stroke by 20 percent. Possible reasons include the fact that fruits and vegetables are rich in antioxidants, potassium, and folic acid, which help prevent oxidation of LDL (bad) cholesterol, help control blood pressure, and fight blocked arteries. That information is based on a two-decade study of 832 people, ages 45 to 65, by Matthew W. Gillman, M.D., Harvard Medical School.

231

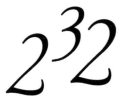

"The greatness of a nation and its moral progress can be judged by the way its animals are treated."

—*Mahatma Gandhi*

232

You may not have to worry about hemorrhoids anymore. It is estimated that at one time or another more than half of all people experience the pain of hemorrhoids. Although they can be caused by heavy physical labor, pregnancy, or prolonged periods of sitting or standing, hemorrhoids are most commonly caused by constipation. When a person is constipated, the simple act of trying to expel matter can cause veins inside or outside the anus to bulge with blood, producing painful hemorrhoids. As common as hemorrhoids are, relief from existing hemorrhoids and preventing future ones may be as simple as adding more fiber to a diet. In fact, ingesting 20 to 25 grams of fiber per day is what most authorities recommend for hemorrhoid relief and prevention. That means eating more whole grain breads, cereals, beans, fruits, and vegetables—exactly the type of foods that most vegetarians consume in abundance.

233

Vegetarianism is a more humane way to live. Canadian author Farley Mowat writes: "If we learn to be compassionate towards other forms of life, we may learn to become compassionate to our own species. We may become humane—at long last."

234

235

You can veg out at Disneyland and Disney World. Veggie burgers are now available at restaurants at both Disneyland and Disney World. The burgers, a product of Fantastic Foods, is on the menu of several restaurants at the Disney theme parks. The same burger will also be appearing soon in the supermarket freezer cases and in other restaurants.

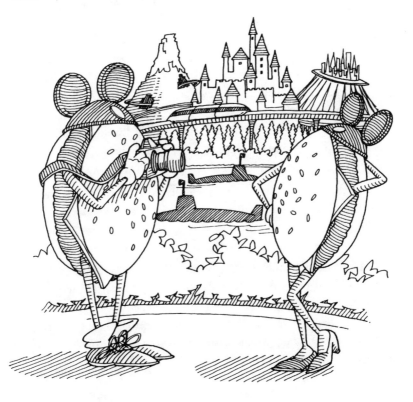

Vegetarians make headlines . . . sometimes. A vegetarian made headlines when he successfully sued a restaurant because his pasta dishes were fishy. Wayne Andrews, a vegetarian for twenty-four years, ate regularly at Pasta Jay's in Boulder, Colorado. He usually ordered pasta with marinara sauce. Then Andrews read in a local paper that his favorite sauce was made with anchovy paste. Upset because the waiters had consistently assured him the sauce was completely vegetarian, he called Pasta Jay's manager. The manager apologized profusely, explaining that the owner concealed the ingredients from the staff.

Using his accounting software, Andrews figured he spent $463.24 on meals at Pasta Jay's. He wrote to owner, Jay Elowsky, requesting a refund. Elowsky countered with an offer of free dinner and drinks for two. Andrews declined and sued Elowsky in small claims court on the grounds that Pasta Jay's had defrauded him by knowingly serving food presented as vegetarian that contained meat. Elowsky argued that "marinara" in Italian means "from the sea," implying the sauce contained fish.

Andrews presented such evidence as a *Webster's* dictionary, which defines marinara as a meatless sauce. Creatively, Andrews also presented the court with several affidavits from Boulder vegetarians describing how waiters at Pasta Jay's told them the marinara sauce was vegetarian, a computer printout detailing his $463.24 worth of meals, and three witnesses who were questioned about his diet. The judge awarded Andrews the total cost of his meals and court fees!

236

"The functioning of the mind is affected by food. There are certain kinds of food that supply the correct material for activating the mental process. Generally speaking, the mind works best on a mild diet, without meat."

237

—*E. R. Rost, British Philosopher*

Vegetarian research helps the Third World. The increasing awareness of the benefits connected to a vegetarian diet helps people in developing countries. Recently, research geneticists in Wisconsin developed a cucumber rich in beta-carotene (beta-carotene is converted into vitamin A in the body). Their hope is that the new cucumber will be grown in developing countries where many children suffer from severe vision problems because they don't get enough vitamin A. Researchers at the Vegetable Crops Research Laboratory in Madison, Wisconsin crossed green cucumbers with those grown in a remote region in China. The hybrid looks like a supermarket cucumber, but its flesh is the color of cantaloupe. Unlike normal cucumbers, which have only a trace of beta-carotene, the new "cukes" have a high amount of beta-carotene. Unlike carrots and melon, cucumbers grow well in hot, humid climates, where most developing nations are located. Also important is the fact that cucumbers retain their nutritional value when pickled. The new cuke will be offered to Third World countries and will soon be in your grocery store, as well.

238

239 *Vegetarians don't contribute to ocean devastation and fish depletion.* The simple fact is that fish are becoming an endangered species as the oceans are plundered to meet human appetite for fish. Decades of mass harvesting from the seas have damaged and even devastated once-rich fishing grounds. Many fishing vessels use $60,000 nets big enough to trap twelve jumbo jets in their quest for fish. Today, there are too many boats chasing fewer and fewer fish. Harvests of cod, haddock, hake, and flounder have dwindled so low in New England, for example, that the federal government has closed several key fishing areas in the hope that near-extinct species will rebound. It remains unclear how fish depletion will affect nature's delicate balances.

240 *You'll be thinking like Lincoln.* Although former President Lincoln may not have been a vegetarian, he made a strong link between animal rights and human rights when he said: "I am in favor of animal rights as well as human rights. That is the way of a whole human being."

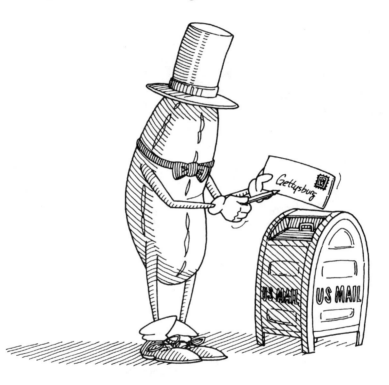

Vegetarianism is consistent with a simple lifestyle. If you, like many others, feel burdened by too many commitments, too little cash, too many possessions, and too little time, and you are tired of keeping up the pace, then you may be ready to consider the rewards of simple living. A good place to start is a vegetarian

241 approach to life. Vegetarianism is very consistent with a simple lifestyle. It recognizes that life can be better when some forms of food are limited or eliminated.

You can let food be your medicine. Many vegetarians are fond of seasoning their food with herbs. Not only do culinary herbs make the food taste better, but many also have several health benefits. Here are a few common culinary herbs that have medicinal benefits:

- *Basil*—Effective in reducing colds, flu, fever, stomach cramps, constipation, headaches, and menstrual pains.
- *Caraway*—These seeds soothe the digestive tract and help eliminate gas.
- *Cinnamon*—Can reduce fever, diarrhea, menstrual problems, and postpartum bleeding.
- *Fennel*—Aids digestion and expels gas. Some studies suggest it may have antibacterial properties.
- *Oregano*—It's good for digestion and acts as an expectorant for coughs, colds, and chest congestion.
- *Parsley*—Research suggests it may be beneficial in treating high blood pressure and in quieting allergy symptoms.
- *Thyme*—Thymol, the active constituent, has antibacterial and antifungal properties and has long been used as an ingredient in mouthwash. Good for treating sore throats, laryngitis, and coughs.

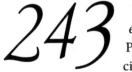

Vegetarians nudge civilization toward another emancipation. Popular radio commentator Paul Harvey notes that progress among civilizations is a series of "emancipations." Vegetarians are an important part of that process. Here is Harvey's insight: "Nature in the raw is cruel—of course it is! Animals can indeed be cruel to one another. But we are supposed to be something more than they! Dickensian compassion rescued children from sweat shops. Lincolnian empathy rescued slaves from being 'things.' Civilization weeps while it awaits one more emancipation."

You'll be one with the Dalai Lama. The Dalai Lama of Tibet makes this observation, with which most vegetarians agree: "Life is as dear to a mute creature as it is to a man. Just as one wants happiness and fears pain, just as one wants to live and not die, so do other creatures."

244

245

Fish is easily contaminated by human waste. Although fish is often the last flesh food given up by some vegetarians, increasing evidence suggests that perhaps it ought to be the first. Recently, the producers of the ABC television program *Prime Time Live* enlisted Nancy Longo to buy fifty pounds of fish from markets in New York, Boston, Chicago, and Baltimore. Longo is an expert at purchasing fish. She owns the Pierpoint, a 44-seat Baltimore waterfront restaurant well-known for its seafood. Longo is a fish aficionado and has sampled more than 275 varieties from around the world, keeping notes on them as if they were fine wines. Each year she buys at least 11,000 pounds of seafood for her restaurant. She loves eating fish, despite suffering an arm infection four years ago that doctors attributed to *Shigella* bacteria in a fish she ate or handled. After Longo made the fish purchases, they were tested for contamination. "20 percent had bacterial levels higher than would be safe for humans to eat. About 40 percent of it contained human fecal matter at a higher level than anyone should consume," she says. The fact is that fish can be easily contaminated by human waste when the seafood is harvested from sewage-polluted waters or when workers don't wash their hands.

Older vegetarian women age better. The average bone loss for female meat-eaters at age 65 is 35 percent. But the average bone loss of female vegetarians at age 65 is only 18 percent.

246

247

"I just don't eat anything that has a mother."
— *Fred Rogers*

Your danger of getting prostate cancer will be minimized. The Harvard Health Letter recently noted that the lowest rate of prostate cancer in the world is among Chinese men living in Shanghai, whose daily food consumption is made up primarily of rice and vegetables. On the other hand, the rate of prostate cancer is much higher among Chinese men in San Francisco. The study strongly suggests that the American meat-oriented diet is a key difference in the rates. Their recommendation for American males: Cut back drastically on meat and increase consumption of lentils, carrots, spinach, and salads.

248

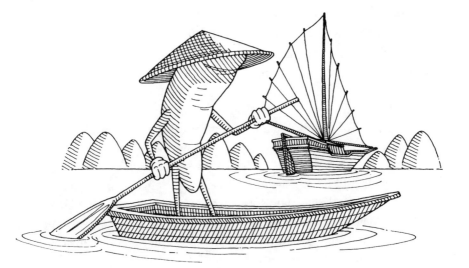

Bart Simpson's sister Lisa is a vegetarian. Approximately 10 million Americans watch *The Simpsons,* one of television's most famous cartoons. In one episode, viewers witnessed Lisa Simpson go vegetarian—with a little help from friends Paul and Linda McCartney. During the episode, Lisa encountered

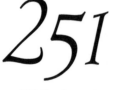 resistance from her brother, Bart, and her father, Homer. However, Lisa prevailed and remained a vegetarian.

Paul and Linda McCartney want to make a believer out of you. The famous Beatle and his wife are well-known vegetarians. They are also eager for their friends and associates to join them in this naturally healthy diet, which protects all animal and sea life. In fact, when David Mirkin, executive producer of *The Simpsons,* flew to Sussex, England to record Linda's and Paul's speaking parts for a *Simpsons* episode at their studio, Linda tried to persuade Mirkin (a sometime vegetarian, who does eat fish) to go vegetarian. "Linda told me, 'It's not seafood, it's sea life'," Mirkin recalls. **250**

251 *The whole Allium family may interest you more.* "What is the *Allium* family?" you're probably wondering. Members of the genus *Allium* include onions, leeks, scallions, and shallots. While the onion—red and vidalia—is common on most plates, vegetarians often develop a fondness for other members of the clan. Not only do they spice up a dish, but the *Allium* genus of foods is very good for the body. Early research indicates that onions, in all forms, may help offset artery-clogging effects of a high-fat diet. Also, certain substances in onions seem to inhibit the formation of blood clots, a principal trigger of most heart attacks. And some studies show that onions may guard against the development of stomach cancer.

252

"Be kind and compassionate to all creatures that the Holy One, blessed be He, created in this world. Never beat nor inflict pain on any animal, beast, bird, or insect. Do not throw stones at a dog or a cat, nor kill flies or wasps."

—*Sefer Chasidim (Ancient medieval Hebrew book)*

253

You can enjoy burgers fresh from the garden. If you're concerned about missing out on eating a hamburger, worry no more. Health food stores, as well as many groceries, now carry delicious, delightful burgers that are entirely meatless. These garden burgers are moist, flavorful, and delicious, especially when augmented with a slice of tomato, onion, and lettuce.

254

Vegetarian meals make the grade at a high school in Maryland. The nutrition science class at Walt Whitman High School in Bethesda, Maryland polled ninety-three students to find out how many were vegetarian. Although only eleven of the ninety-three said they were vegetarians, a whopping seventy-five of ninety-three said that they would purchase a vegetarian option, if it were available in the cafeteria. Armed with this promising response, the nutrition science class, under the direction of their home economics teacher, took on the challenge. The group developed Italian, Chinese, Mexican, Middle Eastern, and American vegetarian-based dishes. Students responded positively to the vegetarian meals, and many were surprised that such tasty recipes could be made without meat. Recipes included Walt Whitman Chili, vegetarian pizza, and tacos with Spanish rice. The end result is that now a vegetarian meal is an option at Walt Whitman High.

It's a good way to meet people. Many vegetarians enjoy dating but are not comfortable paying for others' meals that include meat. Today, most vegetarian magazines carry personal ads through which vegetarian singles can connect with one another. This is a great way to meet people with whom you share common interests.

255

A meatless diet embraces a larger ethic. That certainly was the opinion of Dr. Albert Schweitzer, who wrote the following in his book *Civilization and Ethics:* "My life is full of meaning to me. The life around me must be full of significance to itself. If I am to expect others to respect my life, then I must respect the other

256 life I see. Ethics in our Western world has hitherto been largely limited to the relations of man to man. But that is a limited ethics. We need a boundless ethics, which will include the animals also."

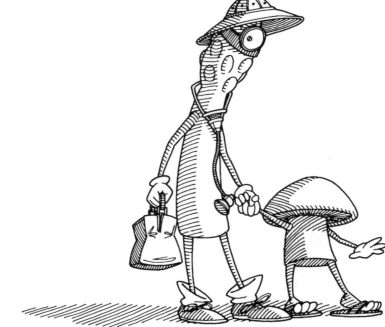

The ASCN believes strongly in a vegetarian diet. "What is the ASCN?" you may be wondering. It is the prestigious American Society for Clinical Nutrition. That group recently released a supplement to its journal espousing the benefits of the Mediterranean diet. The special issue strongly supports a largely plant- and grain-based diet for improved health, adding that such a diet would have a positive impact on agriculture and the environment as well.

257

258 "Moral and legal rules condemning the treatment of animals are based on the principle that animals are part of God's creation towards which man bears responsibility. Laws . . . make it clear not only that cruelty to animals is forbidden, but also that compassion and mercy to them are demanded of man by God. . . . In later rabbinic literature. . . . great prominence is also given to demonstrating God's mercy to animals, and to the importance of not causing them pain. . . . The principle of kindness to animals . . . is as though God's treatment of man will be according to [people's] treatment of animals."

—*Encyclopaedia Judaica*

It's food for the eyes. In a recent study, those who ate spinach or other dark, leafy, green vegetables, such as collard and mustard greens, two to four times a week had healthier maculae (the central part of the retinal layer) and better vision than those who did not. Results combined vegetables of all types—canned or fresh, cooked or raw. According to Johanna M. Seddon, M.D., associate professor of ophthalmology at Harvard Medical School, a possible explanation lies in the fact that these greens are rich in lutein and zeaxanthin, pigments that are vital to vision but can become damaged or destroyed by light and aging.

259

These statistics won't alarm you if you're a female 260
vegetarian. Here are some sobering statistics
concerning women whose diets are primarily
animal-based.

- The increased risk of breast cancer for women who eat meat
  daily compared with those who eat it less than once a week:
  3.8 times.

- The increased risk of breast cancer for women who eat eggs
  daily compared with those who eat them once a week: 2.8
  times.

- The increased risk of breast cancer for women who eat
  butter and cheese three times a week compared with those
  who eat them once a week: 3.2 times.

261 *Raw shellfish is a hazardous food.* That is the
opinion of Mark L. Tamplin, Ph.D., associate
professor of food safety at the University of
Florida in Gainesville. Consider the sad story of a daughter who
took her 80-year-old father out for dinner. The father ordered raw
oysters on the half-shell. Twenty-four hours later, he was dead
after complaining that he wasn't feeling well and was unable to
get out of bed. The cause of death was a comma-shaped shellfish
bacterium called *Vibrio vulnificus.* It is not known how many
people get sick and survive a *vulnificus* infection, but ten to
fifteen people die from it nationwide every year. Experts believe
that *vulnificus* reside in every oyster harvested from areas where
salt- and freshwater mix and the water temperature is greater
than 68 degrees, such as the Gulf of Mexico, the source of most
oysters consumed in the United States. "If you eat a shucked
oyster, you're eating its intestines in a raw form," says Dr.
Tamplin. The risk from the intestinal contents, Tamplin says, is
not just of a *vulnificus* infection but also of hepatitis and
Salmonella.

You'll know the different names for fruits and vegetables wherever you go. Did you know that in the United Kingdom eggplants are called aubergines? Zucchinis are called courgettes in Britain. Raisins go by the name sultanas in other parts of the world.

262

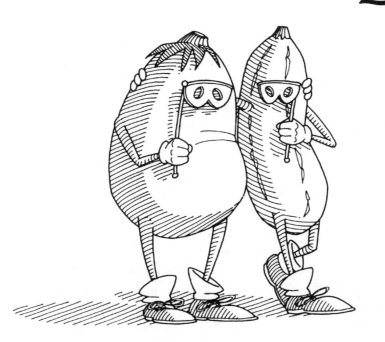

You will be your own "Department of Nutrition." Michael Klaper, M.D., is a physician who believes that people can become well through proper eating. "I am convinced that a proper diet is essential for maintaining or regaining one's physical well-being. Every person is in charge of their own 'Department of Nutrition,' and, given the right guidelines, can make the best choices for themselves." When asked which food choices are most advantageous, Dr. Klaper answers simply: "There is strong medical evidence that complete freedom from eating animal flesh or cow's milk products is a gateway to optimal nutritional health."

263

Meat-based diets have resulted in horrendous animal abuse. Among the many women and men from all walks of life who are expressing concern over **264** factory farming is Janet Hamilton, president of Wilderness Ranch, an organization that helps abused farm animals. "It has been well-documented that the American meat-based diet is causing horrendous animal abuse," she states. "These are feeling, sentient beings enslaved by a system that treats them like car parts."

265 *When vegetarians speak, supermarket executives listen.* Vegetarian Barbara Lovitts of Washington, DC detested receiving coupons for meat from her local Safeway Supermarket. So she wrote a letter to Safeway officials suggesting they survey customers to find out whether they want to receive coupons for meat, or would prefer something else. Although the survey was not done, a few months later, coupons for meat products began to arrive with a new line of small print under the discount offer: "Or your favorite vegetarian alternative." "We had many calls from many customers requesting this option, so we gave it to them," explains Larry Johnson, public affairs director for Safeway's Eastern Division. Lovitts now uses the coupons whenever she can. "My favorite vegetarian alternative is apples," she says.

You will contribute to the health of the nation. Here are some simple but accurate facts:

- World populations with high meat intakes that do not have correspondingly high rates of colon cancer: *none.*
- World populations with low meat intakes that do not have correspondingly low rates of colon cancer: *none.* **266**

These statistics won't alarm you if you're a male vegetarian. Here are some sobering statistics concerning men whose diets are primarily animal-based. Keep in mind that heart disease is the most common cause of death in the United States.

- Risk of death from heart disease for the average American man whose diet is animal-based: 50 percent.
- Risk of death from heart disease for the average American man who consumes no meat: 15 percent.
- Risk of death from heart disease for the average American man who consumes no meat, dairy products, or eggs: 4 percent.

267

268

Your body will thank you by providing you with increased pleasure and health. After John Robbins published his book on the benefits of vegetarianism, *Diet for a New America,* he received more than 30,000 letters from people thanking him. In those letters, many described the benefits they were enjoying as a result of being vegetarians. People reported that their minds became sharper and clearer, their capacities for pleasure and enjoyment had increased, they lost weight, their cholesterol levels were down, they no longer needed the blood pressure medication and diabetes pills that they had been told they would have to take for the rest of their lives, their joints no longer hurt, their sexual functioning returned, they didn't have the headaches or constipation they had previously, and they didn't catch colds or flus as much as they used to.

"You have just dined, and however scrupulously the slaughterhouse is concealed in the graceful distance of miles, there is complicity."

—*Ralph Waldo Emerson*

269

270 *Less is more.* As people eat less meat, there will be more rain forests. A typical 4-ounce hamburger made from rain-forest beef represents the destruction of 55 square feet of tropical forest, an area equal to the size of a small kitchen.

Even dairy products are hazardous to health. During World War I when Norway was occupied by the Germans, Norwegians ate far less meat, eggs, cheese, and cream. Although the death rate from heart disease had been climbing in Norway before the war, it fell during the occupation. After the war, consumption of meat, eggs, cheese, and cream went back up, as did the death rate from heart disease. **271**

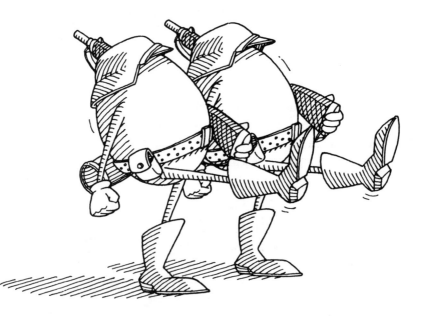

272

Your heart will say "thank you." It is well documented that reduction in meat consumption decreases the risk of heart disease. Here are some impressive statistics:

- Amount you reduce your risk of heart disease with a 10-percent reduction in your consumption of meat, dairy products, and eggs: 8 percent.
- Amount you reduce your risk of heart disease with a 50-percent reduction in your consumption of meat, dairy products, and eggs: 45 percent.
- Amount you reduce your risk of heart disease by eliminating your consumption of meat, dairy products, and eggs: 90 percent.

273

For men, vegetarianism is a natural prostate protector. Men who love their pizza and spaghetti may not only be pleasing their taste buds, they may also be protecting their prostates. As men age, the risk of prostate cancer increases. However, a five-year study of 47,849 men found that those who ate the most cooked tomato products were the ones with the lowest risk of prostate cancer, according to a report published in the *Journal of the National Cancer Institute*. Men who ate ten servings a week of cooked tomato products (one serving is only a one-half cup of tomato sauce or one slice of pizza) had one-third of the risk that men getting only one-and-a-half servings a week had. What is believed to be unique about the tomato's benefit is that it is high in a carotenoid called lycopene. Researchers speculate that lycopene may help prevent cancer from happening by neutralizing free radicals, which can turn innocent cells into cancerous ones. Furthermore, researchers believe that the health benefit of lycopene, the cancer-preventive carotenoid in tomatoes, may be twice as potent as the highly popularized beta-carotene.

You'll feel better. Several years ago, Stephanie Sudden was in a car accident. She required a jaw operation, which forced her to subsist mainly on vegetable and fruit juices. In spite of the accident and eating through wired-shut jaws, Sudden noticed how much better she felt after being forced to give up meat. She subsequently became a vegetarian. Always interested in cooking, Sudden also began to explore vegetarian ways of preparing creative feasts.

274 Today, she is an extremely popular vegetarian chef in the Atlanta area where she prepares meals for private clients and an area restaurant.

Pepper power—nutrition in many colors. Here's a quiz for you—which vegetable has three times as much vitamin C as an orange? Answer: the pepper. Most people are surprised to learn that peppers (a favorite of many vegetarians) are excellent sources of many essential nutrients, especially vitamin C. Green bell peppers have twice as much vitamin C as citrus fruit, red peppers have three times as much vitamin C as citrus fruit, and hot peppers contain even more vitamin C—*357 percent more than oranges!* Also, hot peppers have been reported to increase the blood's ability to break up potentially dangerous clots. And chilies help burn calories by boosting post-meal metabolism. **275**

276 *You can correct people who declare that vegetarianism is a "drastic" lifestyle.* It's ridiculous to believe that changing one's diet to one based on healthy, nutritious, plant-based foods is "drastic." Dr. Dean Ornish puts it into perspective with this observation: "I don't understand why asking people to eat a well-balanced vegetarian diet is considered drastic, while it is medically conservative to cut people open or put them on powerful cholesterol-lowering drugs for the rest of their lives."

277

You can still have "chicken" soup.
Vegetarians quickly find creative ways to simulate some of their favorite flavors. Those who love chicken soup are pleasantly surprised to find that chick peas combined with onions make a soup that tastes and smells almost identical to chicken soup.

New recipes for vegetables don't taste like they're good for you—they just taste good. More and more research indicates that cruciferous vegetables have earned their reputation as disease fighters. Among the protective benefits of crucifers are the blocking of the growth of tumors from cancer-causing toxins, the ability to protect the body from tobacco- and industrial-related cancers, and the inhibiting of some forms of breast cancer by increasing the activity of enzymes that alter estrogen metabolism. Because of that scientific research, more and more recipes are being developed for vegetables from the cruciferous family—cabbage, cauliflower, broccoli, Brussels sprouts, kale, rutabagas, turnips, Swiss chard, and collard and mustard greens. So, unlike those Brussels sprouts you may recall from childhood, the new recipes don't taste like they're good for you—they just taste good.

278

The Santa Fe Opera Company dines on vegetarian fare. **279**
Composers, directors, designers, stars, apprentices,
and technicians of the Santa Fe Opera regularly
dine on vegetarian delights. Their chef, Marsha Chobol, has
always been interested in healthful eating and has recently been
receiving more vegetarian requests. The 500 opera employees
who dine in Chef Chobol's cafeteria include well-known
vegetarians soprano Sheri Greenwald and former executive
director Nigel Redden. Not only is Chobol's salad bar extremely
popular—it's piled high with fresh vegetables, tabbouleh,
couscous, and pasta—but vegetarian sandwiches and entrees,
ranging from simple chili to sophisticated Italian, Indian, Thai,
and other ethnic dishes have also proven to be popular.

280 "Love all God's creating, the whole of it and
every grain of sand. Love every leaf, every
ray of God's light! Love the animals, love
the plants, love everything. . . . Love the animals: God has given
them the rudiments of thought and untroubled joy. Do not,
therefore, trouble them, do not torture them, do not deprive
them of their joy, do not go against God's intent."
                                    —*Feodor Mikhailovich Dostoyevsky*

King Kong-size benefits come in small doses. A recent study of 832
men suggests that males who raise their fruit and vegetable
intake by three servings a day may also be reducing their risk of
stroke by 22 percent. Also the study, published in the *Journal of
the American Medical Association,* noted that an
additional three servings daily might be enough **281**
to trounce any man's risk of stroke. So
vegetarian fare produces King Kong-size
benefits in fairly small doses.

282 Factory farming is producing infections resistant to penicillin. In 1960 only 13 percent of staphylococci infections were resistant to penicillin. In 1988 that number jumped to 91 percent, meaning that penicillin now has very limited impact on staphylococci infections. The major cause for that change has been the breeding of antibiotic-resistant bacteria in factory farms caused by the routine feeding of antibiotics to livestock. In fact, 70 percent of penicillin produced in the United States is used as feed additive in factory farms.

"Until he extends the circle of his compassion to all living things, man will not himself find peace." *283*

—*Albert Schweitzer, M.D.*

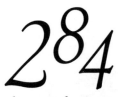 *284* You may discover the fruit that packs the most cancer-fighting beta-carotene. People who adopt a vegetarian diet often quickly discover the mango. Although many Americans still consider the mango an exotic fruit and hesitate to try it, in many tropical countries the mango is as widely consumed as the apple is in North America. Mangoes originated in Southeast Asia, and India is the primary producer of the fruit. Mangoes have 50-percent more beta-carotene than does an equal-sized serving of apricots, and 21-percent more than does cantaloupe. They are popular with many vegetarians, not only because of the cancer-fighting nutrients, but also because the soft, juicy flesh provides a delightful taste sensation—somewhat like a mix of peach and pineapple, only sweeter than either.

285

You will experience tears of joy. A staple in most diets, but especially a vegetarian one, is the onion. It is the one food that cooks cannot imagine cooking without. Yes, they give off a strong odor. Yes, they make some people cry. And, yes, they can linger on the breath. But onions are very, very good for you. They are virtually fat-free and low in calories. At the same time they are very high in fiber; vitamins A, B, and C; calcium; and potassium. They also contain oils that lower LDL levels, or "bad" cholesterol, while raising HDL levels, or "good" cholesterol. If onions make you weep, those tears may be tears of joy; however, here's a tip to prevent the tears when cutting an onion: Try peeling onions under cold, running water and wipe your cutting board with a little white vinegar before chopping. This technique prevents crying when handling onions for many people.

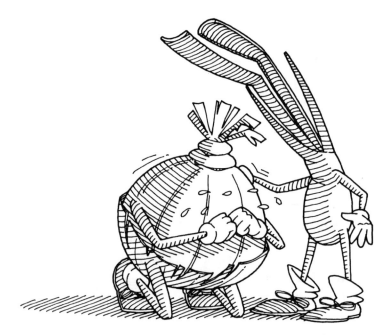

You won't poison your arteries. Animal fat is the dietary demon in heart disease. Populations whose diets are high in animal fat have the highest rates of coronary heart disease in the world. A 1990 World Health Organization report notes that people who eat from 3 to 10 percent of their total calories in animal fat have little heart disease. In the United States and other Western countries, the heart disease rate is much higher and corresponds to a diet rich in saturated fat. Most Americans consume 15 to 20 percent of their calories in animal fat. The lesson is clear: As the intake of animal fat goes up, so does heart disease. "If I had to tell people just one thing to lower their risk of heart disease, it would be to reduce their intake of foods of animal origin, specifically animal fats, and to replace those fats with complex 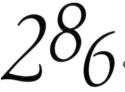 carbohydrates—grains, fruits, and vegetables," advises Ernst Schaefer, M.D., of the USDA Human Nutrition Research Center on Aging at Tufts University.

A lousy diet can make for lousy brain performance. Ketchup stains on your dashboard; hamburger grease on your car seat—there is evidence that a drive-thru diet may not only be messing up your car interior (along with your arteries). It may be messing with your mind as well, according to a study published in *Environmental Health Perspectives.* When fifteen people ate fast food (made up of chicken and mashed potatoes) for two months, they found themselves low in a nutrient called boron. And that lack of boron appears to sap some brainpower. In tests of memory, perception, and attention, the low-boron brain performed less well than when it was recharged with boron. Readings of the brain showed the low-boron state to be closer to drowsiness than to alertness. Many fruits and vegetables are rich in boron.

You may help prevent the demise of Western civilization. It has been noted that the historic cause of the demise of many great civilizations was topsoil depletion. It is amazing and frightening to note that the amount of American topsoil depletion directly associated with livestock-raising is an astounding 85 percent.

288

You can say "salud!" and mean it! The word "salad" comes from the Latin *salus,* meaning "to bring health." Other terms stemming from the same root word include "salubrious" (promoting healing), "salubrity" (wholesomeness), and "salutary" (contributing to some beneficial purpose). And, of course, there is the popular toast, "salud!" meaning "to your health."

289

You will help save the penguins. It's shocking, but the number of penguins at the Punta Tombo wildlife reserve in southern Argentina has dropped by 37 percent over eight years—21 percent during one year alone. The decline is linked to fish consumption by humans, officials say. Huge catches of anchovy, squid, and cod in the South Atlantic during the penguins' breeding season may be to blame, declares Nestor Garcia, director of Wildlife Conservation of Chubut, a region in Argentina. "Once they were killed off by oil spills, and now they are dying of hunger—both problems caused by man," Garcia said.

290

Vegetarianism is a way of reforesting. It is estimated that 35,000 square feet of American land could be returned to forest for each American who adopts a meat-free diet.

291

According to legend, you might survive a snakebite. In the third century AD, the Romans believed that the lemon was an antidote for all poisons. A popular tale of the day involved two criminals thrown to venomous snakes. The one who had eaten a lemon beforehand survived the snakebite, the other died. So great was the reputation of the lemon in Roman times that legend claims it became an accompaniment to fish in the belief that if a fish bone got stuck in the throat, the lemon juice would dissolve it.

The truth is that lemons are very high in vitamin C. Both lemons and limes gained fame for their ability to prevent scurvy, the "curse" of sailors who often went months without fresh fruits and vegetables. Scurvy is a dreaded, potentially fatal, vitamin C-deficiency disease. Muscles waste away, wounds don't heal, bruises appear, and gums bleed and deteriorate. For years, British ships were required by law to carry enough lemon or lime juice for each sailor to have an ounce daily after being ten days at sea. That's why the English are nicknamed "limeys."

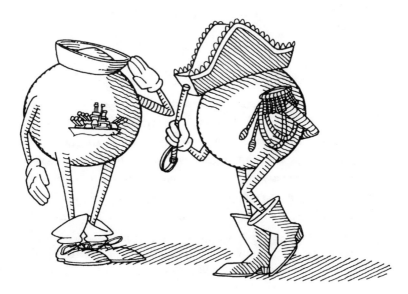

293

You may learn healthier eating habits from other cultures. Vegetarians are often interested in other vegetarians and learn from each other. Here's some information about the eating habits of many in Asian cultures that can guide you to even healthier eating habits.

- Rice and vegetables are the focus of the dishes of many Asian cultures. Steamed or boiled rice (without added fat) dominate most meals.

- They eat more calories, but less fat. Amazingly, the Chinese actually eat more total calories than do Americans—about one-third more. Yet their fat intake is much lower, averaging 14 percent of calories from fat in rural China compared with an average of almost 35 percent of calories in America.

- Fried foods are garnish. Unlike North America where fried foods (which are very high in fat) are popular main dishes, Asians use some fried foods, but only as a garnish.

- They sip soup. In Burma, most don't buy soft drinks, instead they delight in sipping clear, lukewarm broth with meals. The soup, low in fat, acts as a filler that satisfies the appetite.

294

Arsenic. Hog farmers and poultry producers routinely use arsenic as a growth stimulant, despite its carcinogenic properties. Amazingly, federal law allows farmers and producers to use arsenic. However, the government stipulates that livestock owners must discontinue using arsenic in the animals' feed five days prior to slaughter, so that arsenic residue levels will drop to meet FDA standards of .55 ppm (parts per million). However, several studies indicate that livestock producers simply do not comply with this directive. The USDA estimated that nearly 16 percent of the nation's poultry contained residues of arsenic, an amount that exceeds the legal limit.

"I, for my part, wonder of what sort of feeling, mind, or reason that man was possessed who was first to pollute his mouth with gore, and allow his lips to touch the flesh of a murdered being; who spread his table with the mangled form of dead bodies, and claimed as daily food and dainty dishes what but now were beings endowed with movement, with perception and with voice."

—Plutarch

295

You can help the state of California. One of California's leading environmental problems is drought. Listed below are the amounts of water used in California to produce one edible pound of each of the following:

296

- Tomatoes   23 gallons.
- Lettuce   23 gallons.
- Potatoes   24 gallons.
- Wheat   25 gallons.
- Carrots   33 gallons.
- Apples   49 gallons.
- Eggs   544 gallons.
- Chicken   815 gallons.
- Pork   1,630 gallons.
- Beef   5,214 gallons.

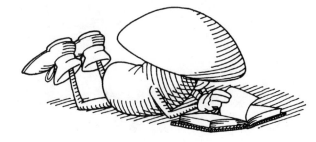

You can tell people the difference between an herb and a spice.
Vegetarians often like to "spice up" their vegetable dishes with
herbs and spices. But do you know the difference between the
two? Herbs are the aromatic leaves, stems, and flowers of plants
that are grown in temperate regions. Examples are basil, thyme,
and oregano. Spices are the aromatic products of the seeds, buds,
fruit, flowers, bark, or roots of plants that are
grown in more tropical regions. Pepper,
cinnamon, and nutmeg are common spices.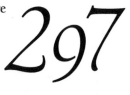

A vegetarian diet can help keep you on your toes. At least that's
true for ballerina Romy Karz, a performer in the Los Angeles
Ballet. As a professional ballerina, Karz dances up to twelve
hours a day, six days a week. She faces a grueling twenty-week
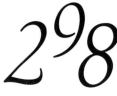 tour each fall and winter. A vegetarian since
the age of seven, Karz links her strength to
her diet: "I have a lot of stamina and
energy," she says.

299 *You won't be part of those who divert food from the hungry.* "The American fast-food diet and the meat-eating habits of the wealthy around the world support a world food system that diverts food resources from the hungry," declares Dr. Walden Bello, executive director of the Institute for Food and Development Policy. "A diet higher in whole grains and legumes and lower in beef and other meat is not just healthier for ourselves, but also contributes to changing the world system that feeds some people and leaves others hungry."

300 *You could save the life of a child.* Currently, a child on earth dies as a result of malnutrition every 2.3 seconds. If more people became vegetarian, there would be an impact on that tragic statistic. Consider these figures:

- Amount of American corn consumed by people: *20%*
- Amount of American corn consumed by livestock: *80%*
- Amount of American soybeans consumed by people: *10%*
- Amount of American soybeans consumed by livestock: *90%*

301 *Raising livestock is a major energy drain.* Not only does the raising of livestock create environmental problems, but it is a major drain of energy sources. "American feed for livestock takes so much energy to grow—counting fuel for farm machinery and for making fertilizers and pesticides—that it might as well be a petroleum by-product," says Alan Durning of the Worldwatch Institute.

Diet is the major factor in health. Former Surgeon General of the United States C. Everett Koop declared: "Your choice of diet can influence your long-term health prospects more than any other action you might take."

302

303 "People often say that humans have always eaten animals, as if this is a justification for continuing the practice. According to this logic, we should not try to prevent people from murdering other people, since this has also been done since the earliest of times."

—*Isaac Bashevis Singer*

You can enjoy angels on your tongue. According to the Irish, potatoes are like "angels on yer tongue." Often referred to as "earth apples" or "spuds," the lowly potato, a national fixation for Americans, is a nutritional powerhouse. High in fiber, vitamin C, complex carbohydrates, and iron and other minerals; a whole pound of potatoes has the same amount of calories as a 4- or 5-ounce hamburger. However, in a potato there is none of the fat found in a hamburger. Of course, the key to keeping the potato an "angel on yer tongue" and not a demon in the body is to avoid the high-fat trappings. Don't fry them or load them up with fatty cheese and sour cream.

304

305 How you eat can lead to wholeness. Author Ashley Montague makes an observation worth thinking about deeply: "Our wholeness as human beings depends upon the depth of our awareness of the fact that we are a part of the wholeness of nature."

Your diet will be just like the chief rabbi's of Israel. Abraham Isaac Kook, the first chief rabbi of the modern state of Israel was a strict vegetarian, as was Scholomo Goren, a recent chief rabbi. Kook's successor, the late Isaac ha-Levi Herzog, promoted vegetarianism. He wrote: "Jews will move increasingly to vegetarianism out of their own deepening knowledge of what their tradition commands. . . . Man's carnivorous nature is not taken for granted or praised in the fundamental teachings of

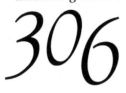

Judaism. . . . A whole galaxy of central rabbinic and spiritual leaders . . . has been affirming vegetarianism as the ultimate meaning of Jewish moral teaching."

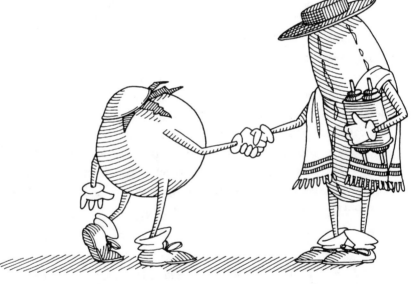

"It must be honestly admitted that, weight for weight, vegetable substances, when they are carefully selected, possess the most striking advantages over animal food in nutritive value. I should like to see the vegetarian and fruit-living plan brought into general use, and I believe it will be."

—*Sir Benjamin W. Richardson, M.D.*

Vegetarianism is a gentle form of social protest. If you're not comfortable marching with a group to protest injustice, take heart. Vegetarianism provides you with a low-key way to make some important points. "To be a vegetarian is to disagree—to disagree with the course of things today," wrote Isaac Bashevis Singer. "Starvation, world hunger, cruelty, waste, wars—we must make a statement against these things. Vegetarianism is my statement. And I think it's a strong one."

308

You can have health insurance in a pod. Many nutritionists refer to the soybean as "health insurance in a pod." Their reasons are compelling. The soybean is the only member of the bean family that contains the proper proportion of all eight essential amino acids, together recognized as a complete protein. The soybean is also rich in B vitamins, calcium, and omega-3 fatty acids, which play an important role in reducing blood clotting, resulting in decreased risk for strokes and heart attacks. Recent research also indicates that soy foods may play a vital role in lowering blood cholesterol; protecting against ovarian, prostate, and breast cancer; and reducing osteoporosis. Vegetarians commonly consume soy products in the form of cooked soybeans, soy flour, soy milk, and tofu.

309

310

It is a cholesterol-free diet. Not a single fruit or vegetable has any cholesterol. Cholesterol comes only from animal sources. A vegetarian-based diet reduces cholesterol in the body. One study revealed that when large amounts of oat bran (slightly more than 1 cup daily), eaten in the form of hot cereal or muffins, were taken by men with high blood cholesterol levels, their readings dropped an impressive 20 percent. One-half cup of cooked beans incorporated into a soup or side dish produced the same results.

You can help feed the American homeless. Because vegetarian food is the healthiest diet for all people, there is an organization dedicated to providing the same vegetarian diet to the homeless. Food Not Bombs, an organization founded in 1980 by a handful of antinuclear activists in Cambridge, Massachusetts, has grown into a network of more than seventy nonprofit chapters nationwide. All of the groups have the same goal: to recover unused vegetarian food from restaurants and natural food stores and offer it, free of charge, to the homeless. Keith McHenry, one of the organization's founders, says that Food Not Bombs, not only provides meals for the homeless, but it educates the general population about food distribution: "We want people to make the connection between vegetarianism and feeding the homeless and hungry," he says. "There is an abundance of food; it is just mismanaged. We really believe in the diet for a small planet." **311**

312 "The indifference, callousness, and contempt that so many people exhibit toward animals is evil, first because it results in great suffering towards animals, and second because it results in an incalculably great impoverishment of human spirit."

—*Ashley Montague*

You will eat like America's first settlers. Robert Beverly, in his book *The History and Present State of Virginia*, published in 1705, provided this information about the diet of America's first settlers: "This Indian corn was the staff of food, upon which the Indians did ever depend. . . . This, with the addition of some peas, beans, and such other fruits of the earth as were then in season, was the families' dependence, and the support of their women and children." **313**

You can help provide vegetarian aid internationally. # 314
Again, because a vegetarian diet is so nutritionally
sound, you can help hungry people around the
world to benefit from the same diet. VegFam is the only overseas
aid charity to provide exclusively vegan food to people in
disaster areas. VegFam, administered by the American Vegan
Society, recently provided more than $10,000 in vegetarian food
aid to civil war victims in Angola, to orphans in India, and to
Rwandan refugees in Tanzania.

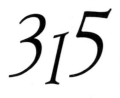

"It is my view that the vegetarian manner of
living, by its purely physical effect on the
human temperament, would most beneficially
influence the lot of mankind."

—*Albert Einstein*

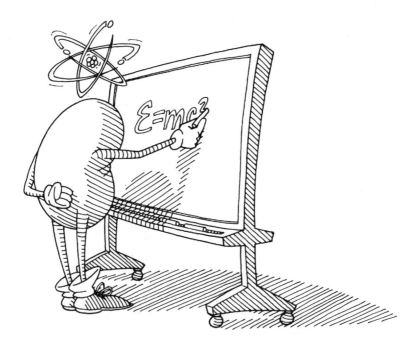

Light delight. As has already been mentioned, because a vegetarian diet is naturally low in fat, it is much easier to lose weight and/or maintain a more slender figure as a vegetarian. Consider British playwright George Bernard Shaw, a vegetarian for nearly seventy years. Shaw relished good food and was well-known for his sweet tooth. He ate massive quantities of cakes, pastries, and honey, yet managed to stay ever-slender and lived to be 94. Of course, no one is recommending that you eat vegetarian so that you can consume huge amounts of desserts, but the fact is that a vegetarian diet is a light delight that allows some people to truly enjoy desserts without major weight gain. *316*

Your children can have a vegetarian pen pal. A vegetarian young person between the ages of 10 and 20 can browse through listings for other vegetarian youths from around the world and establish a pen-pal relationship. Contact The Vegetarian Youth Pen-Pal Directory c/o The Vegetarian Youth Network, P. O. Box

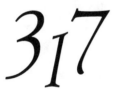

1141, New Paltz, NY 12561. Youths can ask for a registration form and listings. Include a large business-size, stamped, self-addressed envelope for reply.

You could have broken bread with da Vinci. *318* Although Leonardo da Vinci was fascinated with military machinery, he was a vegetarian whose eating habits made him a deeply compassionate man. His love of animals is cited as the reason for his dietary convictions. Legend has it that he bought caged birds just to set them free. In his *Notes*, da Vinci wrote: "I have from an early age abjured the use of meat, and the time will come when men such as I will look upon the murder of animals as they now look upon the murder of men."

Your food won't make you sick. 85 million pigs are slaughtered annually to satisfy the American appetite for ham, pork chops, bacon, etc. Approximately 30 percent of all pork products are contaminated with toxoplasmosis, a disease caused by parasites that can be passed on to consumers.

319

320 If [man] is not to stifle human feelings, he must practice kindness toward animals, for he who is cruel to animals becomes hard also in his dealings with men. We can judge the heart of man by his treatment of animals."

—*Immanuel Kant*

You can eat at colleges. Good news for any vegetarians who plan to attend the world-famous University of California at Berkeley— during the last decade, Berkeley has been dishing up vegetarian meals. Most recently, the school expanded its vegetarian offerings because more and more students requested even more vegetarian options. The offering of vegetarian fare is increasing at college and university campuses across the country.

321

You don't sacrifice the lamb. Great Britain's leading vegetarian researcher is Dr. Alan Long. His many scientific contributions to a better understanding of the benefits of vegetarianism include a twelve-year study of vegetarian health, done in collaboration

322 with Oxford University. Long says he became a vegetarian at age eight because he "preferred the lamb in the field to the lamb on the plate."

Like the West Germans, you will enjoy better health with a vegetarian diet. A recent study done in what was formerly West Germany provides this exciting case for vegetarianism. A five-year study of 1,900 German people who classified themselves as either strict vegetarians (no fish, poultry, meat, or eggs) or moderate vegetarians (some eggs and dairy products with occasional amounts of fish) revealed that these people enjoyed a better level of health and longer life spans than nonvegetarians. Specifically, vegetarians experienced only one-third of the deaths 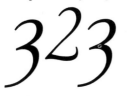 from heart disease that would normally have been expected. Also, they suffered half the expected number of deaths and diseases related to respiratory and digestive disorders.

The Golden Arches may lead to the Pearly Gates. Here's a thought worthy of more reflection: "When you see the Golden Arches, you are probably on the road to the pearly gates," says William Castelli, M.D., director of the Framingham Heart Study.

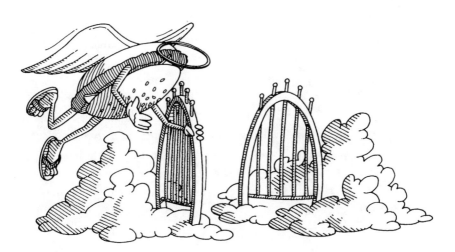

325 *You can prove to your friends that a meal can be filling without being fattening.* Many people, especially men, find it hard to believe that a vegetarian meal can be filling. The truth is that most vegetarian meals are filling without being fattening. If some of your friends are skeptical, treat them to a hearty meal like cream of leek and asparagus soup, roasted potatoes and tomatoes, string beans and walnuts, corn, homemade whole wheat or rye bread, and fruit salad. It will be nutritious, filling, and nonfattening.

You can stay at the Ritz-Carlton. After consulting with experts in nutrition and vegetarian cooking, the Ritz-Carlton Hotel chain has developed **326** exquisite vegetarian meals, now available at the company's 31 resorts and hotels. Ritz-Carlton officials say they developed the new menus in response to customer request—another sign of the impact of the growing vegetarian movement.

327 *You'll be following Puritan beliefs.* Although the United States has been one of the last Western countries to enact basic humane slaughter and laboratory animal welfare legislation (and, then, only through hard-fought battles), it was the first country to enact animal protection legislation. In 1641, the Puritans included in their first legal code: "No man shall exercise any Tirrany or Crueltie towards any bruite Creature which are usually kept for man's use."

You'll have something to beef about. For the majority of vegetarians, the issue of animal suffering becomes important. Many even get politically involved, taking the time to write to and meet with government officials, expressing their concerns. Well-known radio commentator Paul Harvey says: "Ever occur to you why

328 some of us can be this much concerned with animals' suffering? Because government is not. Why not? Animals don't vote."

"I am more thoroughly convinced than ever that meat eating is not only entirely unnecessary, but is physically harmful, as well as an unspiritual practice."

329

—*John Harvey Kellogg, M.D.*

You won't be looked at as a cannibal. Robert Louis Stevenson, the man who wrote many exciting children's books, noted: "Nothing more strongly arouses our disgust than cannibalism, yet we

330 make the same impression on Buddhists and vegetarians, for we feed on babies, though not on our own."

Vegetarians are an important part of a moral evolution. **331** In Tolstoy's Russia there was a growing vegetarian society. That brought pleasure to the Russian writer because he viewed the vegetarian movement as an indication of a moral evolution. "This movement should bring particular joy to those concerned with bringing about the kingdom of God on earth," he wrote, "because vegetarianism is a sign that the aspiration of mankind towards moral perfection is serious and sincere."

332   *You can celebrate with an authentic Thanksgiving meal.* The first Thanksgiving feast meant eating plenty of corn, beans, pumpkin, squash, berries, nuts, herbs, and maple syrup. For the pilgrims, the holiday began as a celebration of survival, of gratitude to local natives who helped save their lives, and of thankfulness for their first bountiful harvest of lifesaving crops. The first Thanksgiving Day meal was primarily and predominantly vegetarian.

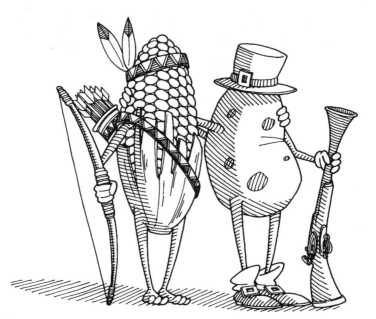

You won't be an accessory to the slaughterhouse. The fact is that animals suffer horribly as they are prepared for slaughter. Author John Updike is more honest than most meat-eaters when he writes: "I'm somewhat shy about the brutal facts of being a carnivore. I don't like meat to look like animals. I prefer it in the form of sausages, hamburger, and meat loaf, far removed from the living thing."

333

334 "The Christian argument for vegetarianism then is simple: since animals belong to God, have value to God, and live for God, then their needless destruction is sinful. In short: animals have some right to their life."

—*Rev. Dr. Andrew Linzey*

You can become the "voice of the voiceless" animals. American poet Ella Wheeler Wilcox (1850-1919) believed human beings had an obligation to speak for the "speechless." She expressed her conviction in this verse: *335*

I am the voice of the voiceless;

Through me the dumb shall speak,

Till the deaf world's ear be made to hear

The wrongs of the wordless weak . . .

And I am my brother's keeper,

And I will fight his fight;

And speak the word for beast and bird

Till the world shall set things right.

A "godlike" sympathy will grow inside of you. Most vegetarians who begin their diets for health or environmental reasons soon develop strong sympathies for animals and their plight. In his book *The Story of My Boyhood*, author John Muir wrote: "Thus, godlike sympathy grows and thrives and spreads far beyond the teachings of churches and schools, where too often the mean, blinding, loveless doctrine is taught that animals have neither *336* mind nor soul, have no rights that we are bound to respect, and were made only for man to be petted, spoiled, slaughtered, or enslaved."

337

You can be vegetarian and a top athlete. An increasing number of world-class athletes are vegetarian. Some notable vegetarian athletes include:

- Stan Price—former world-record-holder in the bench press.
- Robert Sweetgall—former world-record ultra-distance walker.
- Bill Pickering—former world-record-holder for swimming the English Channel.
- Murray Rose—former world-record-holder in the 400- and 1500-meter freestyle swimming.
- Roy Hilligan— winner of the Mr. America body-building championship.
- Pierro Verot—former world-record-holder for downhill endurance skiing.
- Estelle Gray and Cheryl Marek—former world-record-holders for cross-country tandem cycling.
- Ridgely Abele—winner of 8 national championships in karate.

338

"Now what is it moves our very heart, and sickens us so much at the cruelty shown to poor brutes? I suppose this: first, that they have done us no harm; next, that they have not power whatever to resistance; it is the cowardice and tyranny of which they are the victims which make their sufferings so especially touching; . . . there is something so very dreadful, so Satanic in tormenting those who have never harmed us, and who cannot defend themselves, who are utterly in our power."

—*Cardinal John Henry Newman*

339

"Blest is the produce of the trees and in the herbs which the earth brings forth, and the human mouth which was not polluted with blood."

—Ovid

You can eat in the air. Most airlines are more than happy to accommodate a vegetarian. It helps, though, if you let airline officials know ahead of time, so they can prepare a vegetarian meal. In fact, Maxwell Lee, the British-based Hon. General Secretary of the International Vegetarian Union reports that after a series of mix-ups and problems with British Airways regarding vegetarian meals that failed to appear on his flights, he sent a letter detailing the problems to Sir Colin Marshall, the airline's chairman. Soon after, Lee received an apology and a voucher for future travel with British Airways.

340

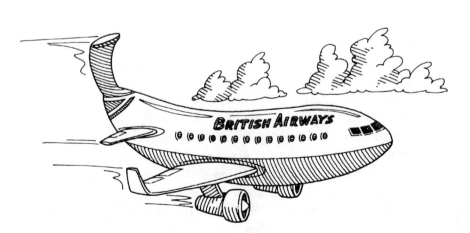

God may not want people to eat meat. There is some **341**
Biblical evidence for the view that God's ultimate
hope is for a world in which no animals are killed, not
even by other animals. One striking example is recorded
by the Jewish prophet Hosea (2:18): "I will make a covenant . . .
with the beasts of the field and the birds of the air and the
creatures that move along the ground. Bow and sword and
battle I will abolish from the land, so that all may lie down in
safety." (New International Version). That statement indicates
the hope of God for a future era in which animals will not be
frightened of capture and death from the bow, the sword, or
other tool of destruction. Other Biblical passages that convey
God's concern for creatures include Genesis 9:9-11, Psalm
145:9, and Isaiah 65:25.

342 *Americans are the most obese people in the
world.* The United States is a country full of
overweight people. "In my experience,
virtually every foreign visitor comments on the number of
overweight people he sees here," says Mona Sutnick, Ed.D.,
R.D., nutritionist and spokesperson for the American Dietetic
Association. "When visitors walk the streets of our cities, they
find it very striking." A stronger, blunter observation is made by
Theodore Van Itallie, M.D., emeritus professor of medicine at
Columbia University's College of Physicians and Surgeons in
New York City: "Americans are among the most obese people in
the world," he says. Even the French—inventors of the high-fat
croissant—are thinner than Americans. The British—eaters of
steak and kidney pie—are also thinner. Northern Europeans—in
spite of their love of ham and cheese—are even thinner. And, of
course, the thinnest people on the planet are Asians, whose diet
is largely vegetarian. Americans would enjoy better health and
thinner bodies if they adopted a vegetarian diet."

343 *You can begin to be truly ethical.* Albert Schweitzer, in his book *The Philosophy of Civilization*, defined a person as "truly ethical only when he obeys the compulsion to help all life which he is able to assist, and shrinks from injuring anything that lives."

344 "Not to hurt our humble brethren [animals] is our first duty to them. But to stop there is not enough. We have a higher mission—to be of service to them wherever they require it."

—*St. Francis of Assisi*

345 *The Talmud teaches compassion for all animals.* Although Judaism teaches that humans are allowed to use and eat animals, the process of slaughter is carefully regulated. The Talmud also warns against a callous disregard of animal welfare. Possibly the most famous Talmudic passage on this teaching is the story of Rabbi Juda (Baba Mezia 85a). A calf was being taken to slaughter, when it broke away and hid its head under the rabbi's skirt, crying out in terror. The rabbi said: "Go; for you were created for this purpose." The response in heaven to the rabbi's indifference was: "Since he has no pity, let us bring suffering upon him." After this, the rabbi suffered from disease for thirteen years. But one day, the rabbi's maid was sweeping the house and was going to sweep away some young weasels lying there. The rabbi said to leave them be, quoting Psalm 145:9—"The Lord is good to all; he has compassion on all he has made." (New International Version). After that incident, the rabbi's heavenly judges relented, and he was healed from his disease.

346

Vegetarianism is a financially sound decision. Most of us enjoy receiving a tax refund from the IRS each year. Switching from a meat-based diet to a vegetarian one offers just such a financial bonus. It has been estimated that a family that consumes meat products adds approximately $4,000 to its annual budget. Although that may not amount to a fortune, any of us, I'm sure, would welcome receiving a surprise check for $4,000. Eric Tyson, author of *Personal Finance for Dummies* even recommends adopting a vegetarian diet as a means of reducing one's cost of living.

Not only do vegetarian foods cost far less than meats, but the body benefits in health terms from them. Vegetarians give their bodies more nutrients, roughage, and vitamins, and less of what hurts the body: chemical additives, saturated fats, hormones, nitrates, and cholesterol.

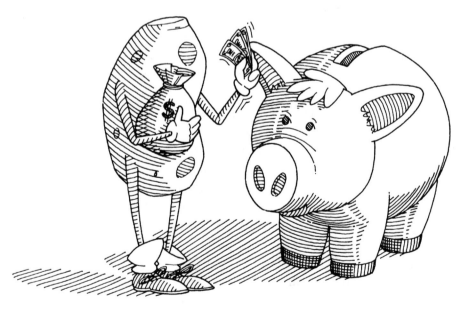

Animals are our equals when it comes to suffering. Peter Singer, the animal rights activist, makes this profound observation in his book *Animal Liberation:* "All the arguments to prove man's superiority cannot shatter this hard fact: in suffering, the animals are our equals."

347

348 *If you want a better world, it's your call.* As has already been noted, today's factory farming is a far cry from farms operated for generations by families, where animals were treated with respect and compassion. Factory farming treats animals as mere pieces of machinery with no regard for their feelings and perceptions. Consider this harrowing account of pigs proceeding to their slaughter by Richard Rhodes who wrote an article for *Harper's Bazaar* magazine titled "Watching the Animals": "The pen narrows like a funnel; the driver behind urge the pigs forward, until one at a time they climb onto the moving ramp. . . . Now they scream, never having been on such a ramp, smelling the smells they smell ahead. . . . It was a frightening experience, seeing their fear, seeing so many of them go by, it had to remind me of things no one wants to be reminded of anymore, all mobs, all death marches, all mass murders and executions." If you want a better world for all creatures, human and animal, it's your call and vegetarianism is an effective way to make that call.

Animals are adorable—"eating bits of them makes no sense." Your cute, playful cat, dog, rabbit, bird, or other pet is adorable. Would you really enjoy cooking up your pet? "We stopped eating meat the day we happened to look out our window during Sunday lunch and saw our young lambs playing happily, as kittens do, in the fields," recalls Linda McCartney. "Eating bits of them suddenly made no sense. In fact, it was revolting."

349

Eating meat is just a cruel habit. In his *Essay on Flesh Eating*, Plutarch, the Greek writer, declared that meat-eating was simply a cruel habit. "Man makes use of flesh, not out of want and necessity, seeing that he has the liberty to make his choice of herbs and fruits, the plenty of which is inexhaustible; but out of luxury, and being cloyed with necessities, he seeks after impure and inconvenient diet, purchased by the slaughter of living beasts; by showing himself more cruel than the most savage of wild beasts."

350 Plutarch's use of the word "inconvenient" is amazingly appropriate now that contemporary research reveals how inefficient it is to produce animals for human consumption.

Vegetarians don't follow the herd. The Roman writer **351** Seneca commended vegetarians for the courage of their convictions and for their individuality. "If true, the Pythagorean principles as to abstaining from flesh foster innocence; if ill-founded they at least teach us frugality, and what loss have you in losing your cruelty? It merely deprives you of the food of lions and vultures. We shall recover our sound reason only if we separate ourselves from the herd. . . . The very fact of the approbation of the multitude is a proof of the unsoundness of the opinion or practice; let us ask what is best—not what is customary. Let us love temperance— let us be just—let us refrain from bloodshed."

352 *A vegetarian world is more just.* Research shows that a vegetarian world could comfortably support several times the current human population. The price of producing one 8-ounce steak could feed up to forty-five or fifty people, each having a full cup of cooked cereal grains. Twenty vegetarians can be fed on the amount of land needed to feed one person consuming a meat-based diet.

The name Luther Burbank will have more meaning for you. In 1940, a three-cent stamp was issued to honor American naturalist and agricultural scientist, Luther Burbank (1846-1926). Born in Lancaster, Massachusetts, Burbank made the planet more attractive and helped its citizens eat better. A century before gene splicing was even heard of, Burbank became the world's best-known plant originator, developing and introducing no less than sixty new varieties of apples, peaches, plums, nectarines, raspberries, and blackberries. In addition, Burbank's' experiments with other edible plants created vastly improved strains of potatoes, tomatoes, corn, peas, squash, and asparagus.

353

"It appears that the first intention of the Maker was to have men live on a strictly vegetarian diet. The very earliest periods of Jewish history are marked with humanitarian conduct towards the lower animal kingdom. . . . It is clearly established that the ancient Hebrews knew, and perhaps were the first among men to know, that animals feel and suffer pain."

354

—*Rabbi Simon Glazer*

"Nothing can be more shocking and horrid than one of our kitchens sprinkled with blood and abounding with the cries of expiring victims or with the limbs of dead animals scattered or hung up here and there."

355

—*Alexander Pope*

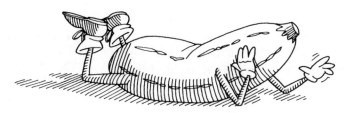

"It is a vulgar error to regard meat in any form as necessary to life. All that is necessary to the human body can be supplied by the vegetable kingdom. It must be admitted as a fact beyond all question that some persons are stronger and more healthy who live on that [vegetarian] food. I know how much of the prevailing meat diet is not merely a wasteful extravagance, but a source of serious evil to the consumer. I have been compelled by facts to accept the conclusion that more physical evil accrues to man from erroneous habits of diet than from even alcoholic drink."

356

—*Sir Henry Thompson, M.D.*

357

You'll do your part to lower this depressing statistic: The appetite for meat in this country appears to be insatiable. To keep pace, the meat industry butchers *14 million animals per day.*

358

A vegetarian diet is superior—period! T. Colin Campbell, Ph.D., is director of the China Health Project, the largest study of diet and health in medical history. He concludes that a vegetarian diet is superior to all other diets. In his words: "I think in the next ten or twenty years, we'll have evidence [showing that a vegetarian diet is superior] that is as strong as the evidence that cigarette smoking causes lung cancer. In my view, it's plenty strong enough now."

"The beef industry has contributed to more American deaths than all the wars of this century, all natural disasters, and all automobile accidents combined."

359

—*Neal Barnard, M.D.*

Your vegetarian diet will show that you are a thinking person.
Consider this observation from Albert Schweitzer, M.D.: "The thinking [person] must oppose all cruel customs, no matter how deeply rooted in tradition and surrounded by a halo. When we have a choice, we must avoid bringing torment and injury into the life of another."

360

361 *You can impress your friends with some useless but interesting facts.* Did you know that the largest fruit ever grown was a 990 lb. pumpkin grown in 1994 in Ashton, Ontario, Canada by Herman Bax? The largest vegetable is a 124 lb. cabbage grown by B. Lavery in Llanharry, Wales in 1989.

Remember, you are a primate, and primates don't eat meat. Dr. Neal Barnard, president of the Physicians Committee for Responsible Medicine, says: "We

362

are primates, and primates are all vegetarians with only rare meat consumption by certain species. All the protein, minerals, and vitamins the human body needs are easily obtained from plant sources. The taste for meats and other fatty foods is like a substance abuse to which we are addicted early in life. While we have been struggling—and failing—to cure heart disease and cancer, their primary causes are right under our noses, on the dinner table."

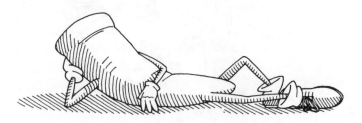

363

"We don't eat anything that has to be killed for us. We've been through a lot, and we've reached a stage where we really value life."

—*Paul and Linda McCartney*

"I feel that spiritual progress does demand at some stage that we should cease to kill our fellow creatures for the satisfaction of our bodily wants."

—*Mahatma Gandhi*

364

365

Factory farming has ended the era of the cowboy. It has been sadly noted that the cowboy is gone. Today's "modern" cowboys don't run 500 heads of cattle on 10,000 acres of open prairie. Today, the "modern" cowboy is likely to run 10,000 head of cattle on 5 acres of concrete.

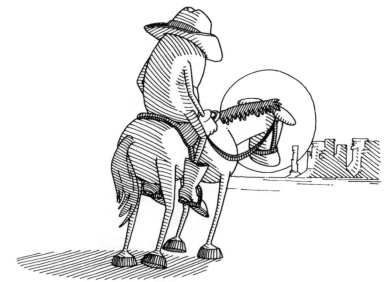

When I began researching and writing this book, I had three types of readers in mind: those who are vegetarian, those who are seriously considering vegetarianism, and those who are mildly curious about a vegetarian diet. If you are a vegetarian, I hope this book has been successful in reinforcing your commitment, has given you additional motivation to remain on the path, and has inspired you sufficiently that you, in turn, can inform others about the many benefits of vegetarianism. On the other hand, if those of you who read the book were simply curious about becoming vegetarians, I sincerely hope the information you read has convinced you to join me and millions of others in this healthy lifestyle. No matter what the reason for your decision to be a vegetarian, your choice will be a wise one. With the passing of time, you will personally discover the benefits of vegetarianism.

Now, I would like to ask you, the reader, to do two things. First of all, if you found this book helpful, perhaps you could pass on your copy to someone else or purchase an additional book as a gift for a friend, who, like you, is interested in vegetarianism. Second, I would like you to write to me in care of the publisher, suggesting additional reasons that you feel are important for being a vegetarian. I will continue to research and file away information. Your thoughts and opinions are important to me. Kindly contact me at this address:

Victor M. Parachin
c/o Avery Publishing Group
120 Old Broadway
Garden City Park, NY 11040

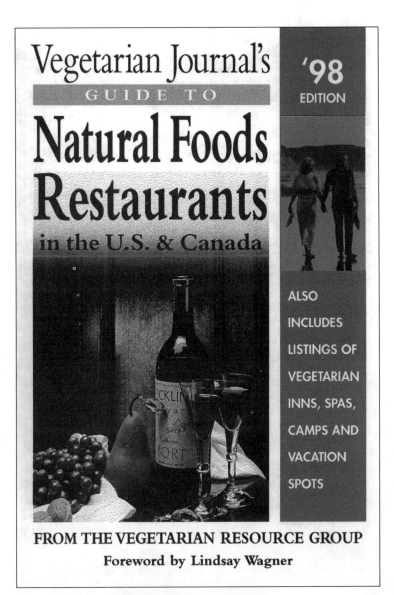

Vegetarian Journal's
GUIDE TO
Natural Foods
Restaurants
in the U.S. & Canada

'98
EDITION

ALSO
INCLUDES
LISTINGS OF
VEGETARIAN
INNS, SPAS,
CAMPS AND
VACATION
SPOTS

FROM THE VEGETARIAN RESOURCE GROUP
Foreword by Lindsay Wagner

0-89529-837-6 • $12.95

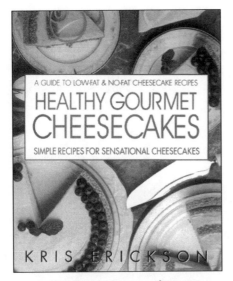
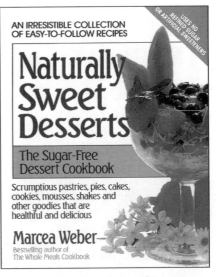
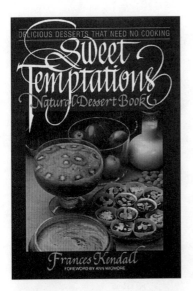
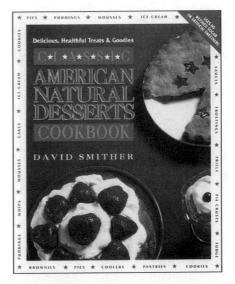

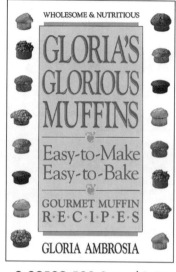
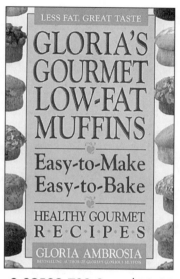
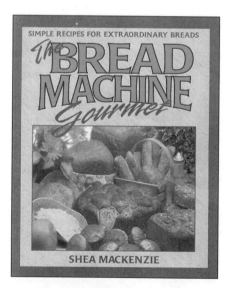
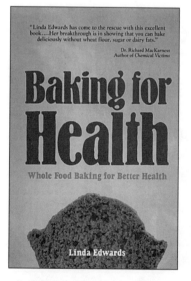

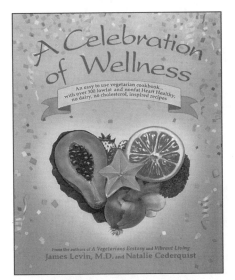

0-89529-684-5 • $17.95

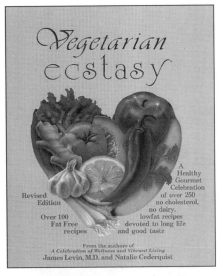

0-89529-682-9 • $16.95

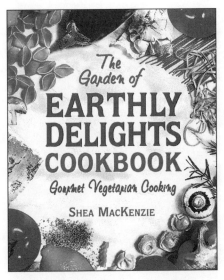

0-89529-530-X • $14.95

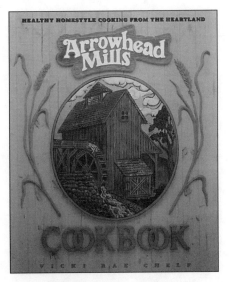

0-89529-546-6 • $14.95

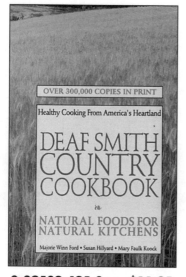
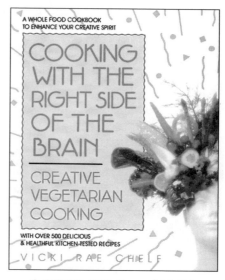
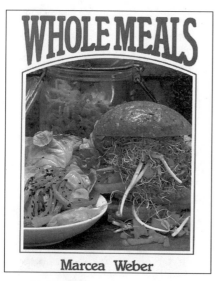
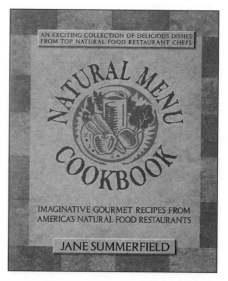

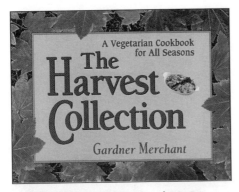

0-89529-615-2 • $12.95

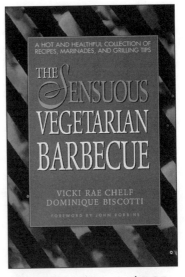

0-89529-613-6 • $9.95

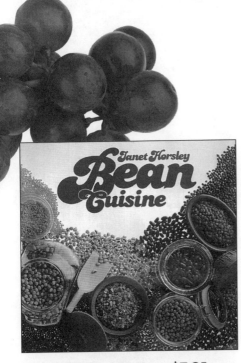

0-89529-446-X • $7.95

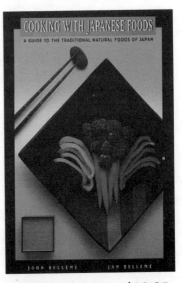

0-89529-583-0 • $13.95

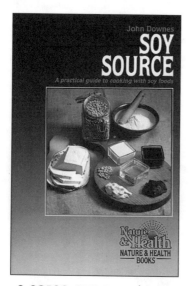
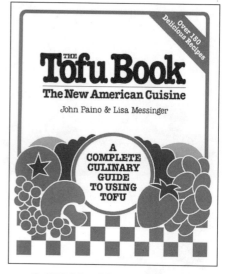
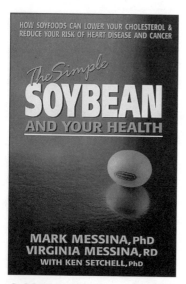
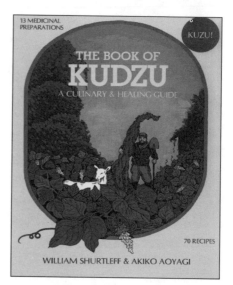

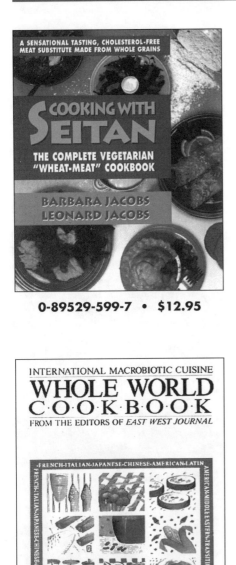

0-89529-599-7 • $12.95

INTERNATIONAL MACROBIOTIC CUISINE

WHOLE WORLD
C·O·O·K·B·O·O·K

FROM THE EDITORS OF *EAST WEST JOURNAL*

0-89529-231-9 • $6.95

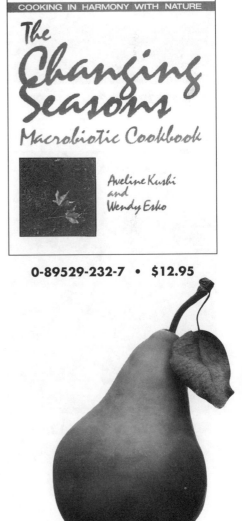

0-89529-232-7 • $12.95

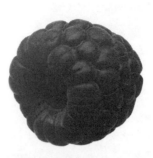

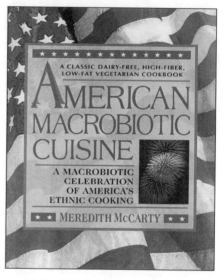

0-89529-442-7 • $11.95

0-89529-711-6 • $12.95

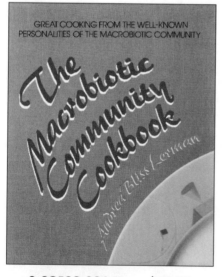

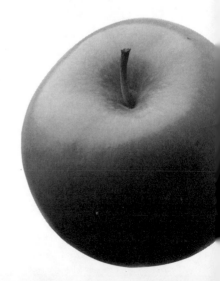

0-89529-396-X • $12.95

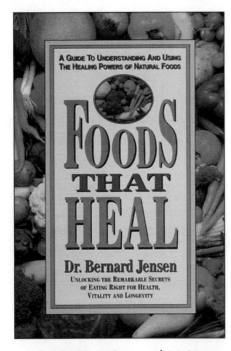
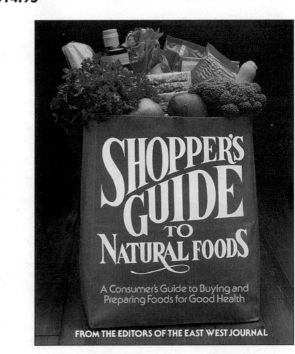

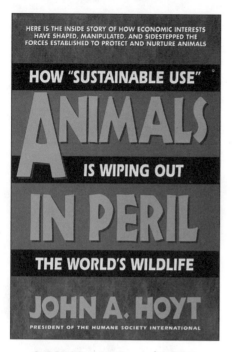
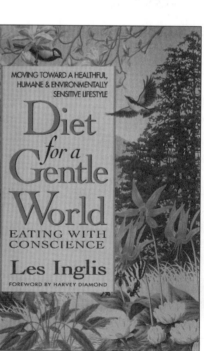
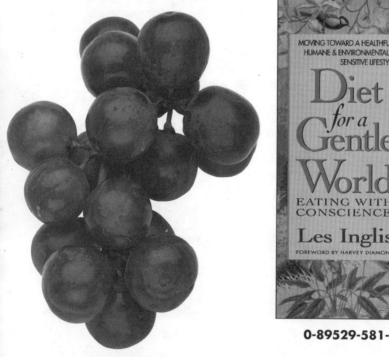